1995

SCIENCE & TECHNOLOGY   *Health Sciences*

33-5131   RA644   94-30389 CIP
Chronic illness: from experience to policy, ed. by S. Kay Toombs, David Barnard,
and Ronald A. Carson. Indiana, 1995. 221p bibl index afp ISBN 0-253-36011-0, $27.95

Toombs, Barnard, and Carson have organized and edited a valuable series of papers that provide a rare perspective on the impact of chronic illness. Beginning with the person who is experiencing the chronic condition, they are able to weave an important blend of personal, social, and policy themes. The fundamental values expressed by health and social service providers, and policy makers who work on behalf of individuals with chronic conditions, underscore the importance of beginning with the person when planning, organizing, and delivering services, or developing state and federal policy. Yet, rarely does that happen in practice or in textbooks and articles that are used to prepare people for practice. This book provides the reader with the opportunity to better understand and reflect upon the opportunities and challenges of daily life as experienced by a person with a chronic condition. It would be a valuable resource for students in health-related studies or the social sciences. General; upper-division undergraduates through professionals.—*M. Richardson, University of Washington*

CHRONIC ILLNESS

MEDICAL ETHICS SERIES

DAVID H. SMITH AND ROBERT M. VEATCH

EDITORS

CHRONIC ILLNESS
From Experience to Policy

EDITED BY

S. KAY TOOMBS,
DAVID BARNARD,
AND
RONALD A. CARSON

WITH CONTRIBUTIONS BY

S. KAY TOOMBS, RUTHANNE L. CURRY, DAVID BARNARD,
LONNIE D. KLIEVER, SUE E. ESTROFF, RONALD A. CARSON,
GEORGE J. AGICH, JOHN W. DOUARD, ARTHUR KLEINMAN,
MURIEL R. GILLICK

INDIANA UNIVERSITY PRESS
BLOOMINGTON AND INDIANAPOLIS

The paper used in this publication meets the minimum
requirements of American National Standard for Information
Sciences—Permanence of Paper for Printed Library Materials,
ANSI Z39.48-1984.
∞™

Library of Congress Cataloging-in-Publication Data
Chronic illness : from experience to policy / edited by S. Kay Toombs,
David Barnard, and Ronald A. Carson.
p. cm. — (Medical ethics series)
Includes bibliographical references and index.
ISBN 0-253-36011-0
1. Chronic diseases—Social aspects. 2. Chronic diseases—
Psychological aspects. I. Toombs, S. Kay, date. II. Barnard,
David, date. III. Carson, Ronald A. IV. Series.
RA644.5.C48 1995
362.1—dc20
94-30389
1 2 3 4 5 00 99 98 97 96 95

In Memoriam,
Irving Kenneth Zola

CONTENTS

❖
———————

PREFACE

THIS BOOK IS devoted to the topic of chronic illness, a topic which has both personal and social relevance. The main diseases of our time—the degenerative diseases of the elderly, cancer, heart disease, AIDS, stroke—are chronic in nature, as are such disorders as multiple sclerosis, persistent mental illness, and diabetes. Since chronic disorders represent the major source of morbidity and mortality in our society with most individuals over sixty experiencing at least one chronic disorder, it is probable that each of us will one day be personally affected, either through our own experience or through that of a family member. Moreover, as a society we face urgent challenges in terms of how best to care for the increasing number of individuals who are chronically ill and disabled, and these challenges must be carefully addressed.

The essays that follow consider a wide variety of issues relating to chronic illness. In particular, they focus upon what chronic illness means to those who are most intimately involved (persons who are ill and those closest to them), as well as deliberating about the implications for social policy, health care, bioethics, and the professions.

Although the essays are grouped in two major sections—the first section focusing primarily on lived experience, the second on ethical, social, cultural, and political responses—it becomes obvious that these dimensions of chronic illness are inextricably interconnected. Indeed, one of the most valuable insights provided by this volume is the recognition that the varying perspectives inform and complement one another in important and unexpected ways.

An adequate exploration of chronic illness must begin with the lived experience (Part One). Before one can properly address issues relating to care, policy, and the appropriate social response to such illness, it is of vital importance to understand its distinctive character. How, for example, does the experience of chronic illness differ from an episode of acute disease? What is it like, how does it feel, to be chronically ill and to live with permanent disability on an everyday basis? What impact does the illness have on an individual's family and on the social world of everyday life? Are there particular sources of suffering for those who are most intimately involved? How can (does) a person with chronic illness rise to meet the challenge? What gives one the strength to endure?

Illness narratives provide a window into the lived experience of chronic illness for those who are not now, not yet, chronically ill or disabled. These narratives, or stories, take different forms. In addition to autobiographical descriptions of chronic illness, such as Kay Toombs' first-person account of what it is like to live with a progressively degenerative disease (multiple sclerosis), there are the stories told by family members. Ruthanne Curry, for instance, narrates the story of an "exceptional" family as she shares the experience of parenting a child with a chronic disability (her son, Robbie, who has cerebral palsy). In addition, there are the narratives recorded by clinicians and ethnographers (which subsequently appear as a component of academic discourse), as well as literary accounts—poems, stories, plays. Illness narratives go far beyond the objective description of a particular disease state. They are not primarily concerned with such matters as elevated blood counts, demonstrable lesions, or abnormal EKGs. Rather, they give voice to the life disruption that illness engenders. In situating illness within the context of a particular life, illness narratives focus on the meaning that illness has for the individual in the midst of everyday life. In so doing, they provide at least an initial response to the question "What is it like to live with chronic illness?"

The stories of illness related in this book disclose certain important themes. The first and perhaps most obvious theme is the embeddedness of the personal narrative in the narratives of others. Since we are social beings, to tell one's own story is necessarily to include the story of others. In addition, the life disruption occasioned by chronic illness engulfs not only the sick person but also the family and other intimates. In this respect, suffering is not only personal, it is interpersonal.

Personal narratives are also necessarily embedded in a social context, a local world. There is a dialectical relation between the individual and society—a constant reciprocity between subjective experiencing and the intersubjective milieu of everyday life. Chronic illness is not only a way of being but a way of *being in the world*. Consequently, just as the illness experience itself influences an individual's capacity to engage the social world, so the social world (societal attitudes, social practices, public policy) influences the subjective experience of illness and its attendant meanings.

The reciprocal relation between self/other, self/society, both motivates the illness narrative and the lived experience and, paradoxically, creates inevitable tensions and ethical dilemmas. To tell one's story is to attempt to convey its significance to others, to call for recognition of one's circumstance. The opportunity to give voice to one's condition to an empathetic listener is a meaningful act in and of itself. At the same time, in the very act of sharing the story, one must unavoidably reveal oneself to the other and thereby risk misunderstanding. This risk is particularly great in the case of a *published* narrative since the other (the audience) is unknown and possibly untrustworthy. As Sue Estroff's essay reveals, this tension is most obvious in the case of chronic illness narrative research, where the ethical dilemmas are particularly acute given the nature of informant-researcher relations. There is also risk involved in giving a first-person, autobiographical account. Although in the latter the sick person speaks for herself and thus hopes to avoid mistranslation, the interpretation of strangers is never predictable. In addition, in the act of telling one's personal story, one is more likely to reflect deeply about the experience. Such personal reflection can force one to face disquieting information about oneself and one's life situation. This is, perhaps, particularly a threat for the chronically ill with mental disorders, many of whom do not readily acknowledge the severity of their illness.

The call for recognition by others on the part of the chronically ill person is a call for empathetic understanding. What is at stake is an attempt to reach the other, to reduce the sense of isolation. The tales told in this book reveal that to live with chronic illness and disability is to experience a sense of "differentness," of loneliness, of rejection, of separation from others, of alienation from society. At the same time, the narratives stress the importance of relationships, of finding others to share the "journey." They speak of the redemptive power of caring and companionship and thus provide important clues as to how to *be with* those who are chronically ill.

A distinctive characteristic of chronic (as opposed to acute) illness is its temporal dimension. Chronic illness persists over time; it does not go away. It is, therefore, not simply a discrete episode in the course of a life narrative but rather a permanent feature of that narrative. To live with chronic illness and disability is to live a certain kind of life. The enduring nature of such a challenge requires a personal and social response that is different in kind from that which is called for by the temporary disruption of acute illness.

Moreover, a much neglected aspect of physical illness is its affective dimension. We experience the world of everyday life not only in terms of physical interaction but in light of our emotions. To ask of the narrative "What is it *like* to be chronically ill or to live with permanent disability?" is necessarily to discover how it *feels*. In exploring the interconnection between the emotions of rage and grief, Lonnie Kliever takes another look at the case of Dax Cowart and considers how this particular case illuminates the experience of suffering in chronic (as opposed to acute) illness. As Dax's story and the other narratives make clear, emotions such as anger, grief, shame, and fear are part and parcel of the everyday experience of ongoing disorder. Indeed, such unavoidable emotions are a principal source of suffering to the disabled and the chronically ill.

Positive emotions such as hope must also be re-examined in the context of chronic illness. In exploring the dynamics of hoping, David Barnard confronts the question of what it can mean to hope in the face of ongoing and permanent disability where cure of disease is not a realistic possibility. Insights from social-psychological and philosophical literature provide important understandings of both the personal and the social dimension of hoping.

Focusing on lived experience forces us to reflect upon ethical, social, and cultural dimensions of chronic illness and disability (Part Two). Personal narratives are necessarily situated in a social world—a world which does much to shape the meaning of the individual's experience. Do the responses we make as family members, caregivers, professionals, and as a society adequately take into account the everyday life of the chronically ill? How is this distinctive experience shaped in the context of our present-day culture? Are there societal values or symbolic meanings which imbue chronic illness with a particular significance? Do certain social practices constrain the chronically ill?

Ronald Carson's essay reveals that poems and stories of chronic sickness and disability cause us to question the adequacy of basic moral principles that currently prevail in bioethics. Insights from such literature motivate a critique of the principle of respect—the cornerstone of contemporary bioethics—as the dominant principle in caring for patients. As traditionally conceived in the context of acute care medicine, the principle of respect (which aims to protect people from violation) does largely negative work. It reminds us to leave one another alone. In the context of chronic illness, however, where a sense of familiarity with a patient's plight and life is imperative in the healing process, too narrow a conception of respect may easily result in the abandonment of patients. The ill are due positive regard (recognition, affirmation, confirmation) as well as negative respect. Additionally, as George Agich points out, standard assumptions about the nature of autonomy prove inadequate in light of the actual day to day experience of chronic illness. In particular, Agich argues that abstract models of autonomy (which focus on freedom from restraint) do not sufficiently take into account the temporal and emotional realities that characterize the life of the chronically ill.

Reflection on lived experience also forces one to recognize the manner in which social attitudes toward chronic illness and disability have an impact on social practices—directly affecting the way people with physical or mental disorders are treated by others, as well as influencing their feelings about themselves and the extent to which they can flourish as members of society. In examining two competing models of disability, John Douard considers in detail the way in which we conceive of, talk about, and classify persons with disabilities, noting how such models not only directly influence the social life of the chronically ill but also determine public policy.

The focus on the dialectical relation between self and society also motivates a critique of the prevailing biomedical interpretation of chronicity. Arthur Kleinman argues that illness exhibits a social (rather than "natural") course. An alternative, ethnographic theory of the relation between the body and its social context reveals that chronic illness unfolds in a social field, or "local world." When we take seriously the social processes that mediate chronic illness, we are forced to question not only the adequacy of the prevailing biomedical model of disease but also the extent to which traditional approaches in bioethics and the medical humanities emphasize the individual experience of illness at the expense of its social and cultural sides.

No consideration of the social dimension of chronic illness would be complete without some reflection on the peculiar challenges it poses to health policy and existing health care systems. These challenges are numerous and include escalating costs, limited resources, issues of long-term care, and availability of care. At the same time, it is of some importance to understand how health policy, in turn, influences care and directly affects the sick person's experience.

The aging of the population in our society is, of course, an important factor when considering health policy for the chronically ill where the care that is provided is largely long-term care. Muriel Gillick provides an analysis of the major institutions providing this care—the nursing home, the rehabilitation hospital, and the home—showing how burgeoning regulations affect both the quality of care (in the technical, medical sense) and the quality of life of those served. Such an analysis suggests the need for reform of the long-term care system if we are to respond adequately to the needs of the chronically ill.

Consideration of the social aspects of chronic illness brings us full circle. Our exploration began with a focus on the individual living with chronic illness in the social world of everyday life. In exploring the narrative we asked how the personal experience can, and should, inform the response of others. In expanding our gaze to the wider social context, we have reflected upon how that response is shaped by, and shapes, the individual experience.

Certain key themes have emerged in the course of this exploration: (1) the importance of narrative and of empathetic attention to the individual voice; (2) the dialectical relationship between the individual and society, and especially the interplay between social, cultural, and political responses to chronic illness and the chronically ill person's actual experience; (3) the opportunity and need to reflect upon, and reconsider, prevailing principles in bioethics and traditional biomedical approaches to illness in light of serious engagement with the lived realities of chronic illness and disability.

The essays in this volume thus provide a clearer understanding of the peculiar challenges that chronic illness and disability pose for us as individuals and as professionals. In particular, they remind us of the necessity of paying heed to the lived experience while, at the same time, responding in such a way as to positively affect that experience.

S. Kay Toombs, David Barnard, Ronald A. Carson

❖
───────────────

ACKNOWLEDGMENTS

THIS BOOK IS the outcome of a year-long project culminating in a two-day dialogue that took place at a collaborative seminar held at the Institute for the Medical Humanities in Galveston, Texas. The participants brought to the dialogue the differing perspectives of medicine, sociology, philosophy, religion, nursing, and the medical humanities. Some of the participants have personal experience of chronic illness, some are professionally involved with the chronically ill as caregivers or researchers, some are engaged in undergraduate or graduate education, and some are involved in the education of health professionals. The project was made possible by the Jesse H. Jones Endowment for Research in the Medical Humanities, established at the University of Texas Medical Branch by awards from the National Endowment for the Humanities Challenge Grant Program and The Houston Endowment.

The editors would like to thank Diane Pfeil for her invaluable assistance in preparing the manuscript for publication.

PART ONE

SUFFICIENT UNTO THE DAY
A Life with Multiple Sclerosis

S. KAY TOOMBS

DISSEMINATED SCLEROSIS: Disseminated, or multiple sclerosis is one of the commonest nervous diseases. It is characterized by the widespread occurrence of patches of demyelination followed by gliosis in the white matter of the nervous system. A striking feature is the tendency to remissions and relapses, so that the course of the disease may be prolonged for many years. The early symptoms are those of focal lesions of the nervous system, while the later clinical picture is one of progressive dissemination. The cause of the disorder is unknown.

There are two chief modes of onset. In most cases the disease begins with the symptoms of a single focal lesion or sometimes of several such lesions occurring within a short time. Unilateral acute retrobulbar neuritis is often the first symptom. Other such symptoms include numbness of some part of the body, usually a part of a limb or one side of the face or both lower limbs, or double vision, or weakness of a limb, particularly of a lower limb with dragging of the foot, or precipitancy of micturation. The other mode of onset is an insidious and slowly progressive weakness of one or both lower limbs.

In the insidiously progressive type of case, the abnormal physical signs are usually predominantly spinal, consisting of spastic paraplegia with some degree of superficial sensory loss over the lower limbs and trunk, or of impairment of postural sensibility and vibrations sense or sometimes of both combined, the patient exhibiting a spastic and ataxic gait. In such cases, it may be difficult to be sure that the symptoms are due to disseminated sclerosis unless there is a history or there are physical signs of lesions within the territory of the cranial nerves, or characteristic changes in the cerebrospinal fluid.

In a typical advanced case, the patient will be bedridden with scanning or staccato speech and slurring of individual syllables, pallor of both optic discs, nystagmus, and a dissociation of conjugate lateral movement of the eyes, the abducting eye moving outwards further than the adducting eye moves inwards. The upper limbs will be weak and grossly ataxic. There will be severe paraplegia, either in extension interrupted by flexor spasms, or in flexion. Cutaneous or deep sensory loss, or both, may be present in upper or lower limbs, and there is likely to be incontinence of urine and feces.

ROGER BANNISTER
BRAIN'S CLINICAL NEUROLOGY

EVERY MULTIPLE SCLEROSIS patient can remember the moment of diagnosis. It is one of those events that can forever be recalled in the most exquisite detail. I can, for example, describe the clothes I was wearing, tell you what day of the week it was (a Thursday), pinpoint the date (almost exactly three months prior to my thirtieth birthday), repeat verbatim the words used by the neurosurgeon, and recollect shivering violently with cold as I came out of the building into the stifling Texas heat. I can also remember wishing fervently that I could go back a few moments in time, for I recognized that the pronouncement of the diagnosis had changed my life in a fundamental way.

For one thing, I was not going to get well—ever. Though I might have periods of remission, I would not (and could not) be cured. My expectation had been that medicine would restore me to health. Now that expectation was dashed, along with my cherished illusion that I was in control of my life. The future disappeared. I could think only of the activities I would no longer be able to enjoy, the work I would have to give up, the disruption that would engulf my family life. I felt an elemental loss of wholeness. My body, which I had always taken so much for granted, was irrevocably flawed. Indeed, no longer to be trusted, it posed a threat to my very existence. Above all, there was the overwhelming realization that, from that point on, I would live every day with uncertainty, never knowing (from one day to the next) what the extent of my physical capacities would be.

My initial response was terror. Just two days earlier, by a strange coincidence, I had read a magazine article about the plight of a young woman with M.S. The photos accompanying the story are still imprinted on my mind. In one, the woman posed coquettishly in a bathing suit with a "Miss Michigan" sash emblazoned across her chest. In the other, she sat dejectedly in a wheelchair, appearing broken and helpless. The author explained that she was paralyzed, unable to care for herself, that her disease was progressive, that treatment was controversial, and that there was no known cure.

Not surprisingly, on hearing my diagnosis, my first question to the physician was, "Will I end up in a wheelchair?" He replied he was sorry but he could give me no guarantees for the future. I interpreted this to mean that I would soon be like the woman in the magazine. (This dire interpretation was reinforced when, on arriving home, I looked up the disease in an outdated edition of an encyclopedia. The entry stated that M.S. was an incurable, progressive disease of the central nervous system culminating in total paralysis and death.)

Of course, in retrospect and with the benefit of nineteen years' experience, I now know that the physician could have answered my question differently. It's not that his response was incorrect. (He could not guarantee my future physical

state—for that matter, who can?) But not *all* M.S. patients end up severely incapacitated and, while there are patients who suffer a rapidly progressive course,
they are in the minority. I wish he had told me that too.

The diagnosis had an equally devastating effect on my husband. At the time,
he was a student attending college on the G.I. Bill. He had two long years to go to
complete his degree. His future suddenly appeared as tentative as mine. I was the
"breadwinner" of the family. Would I be able to continue to work, to support him
in his endeavors? He wondered aloud if he would be forced to abandon *his* goals,
to give up on *his* dreams.

A week or so later, seeking information, we together attended a meeting of the
local chapter of the M.S. Society. Seeing people there in wheelchairs served to confirm our unspoken fears. The worst part of the evening was the movie. The film,
while informational, was obviously primarily intended as a means to raise money
for research. It should never—ever—have been shown to a newly diagnosed patient (or to any patient, for that matter).[1] Entitled "My Friend Joe," it depicted in
detail the rapid physical decline of a young man—once a lively, active, high school
athlete—who was stricken with M.S. in early adulthood. The movie began with
Joe's happy marriage to his high school sweetheart, the subsequent purchase of
their house, the birth of their children, and the blossoming of Joe's career. Then
came the day when Joe experienced the seemingly innocuous symptoms of stum-
bling on the stairs, and dropping a ball while playing with his children. Joe went
to the doctor. Tests were performed. The diagnosis was pronounced. The sentence
was passed. The last scene of the movie depicted Joe in a wheelchair. He had not
aged. Indeed, it seemed that little time had elapsed. He was, however, no longer
vibrant. Apparently unable to move either his arms or his legs, he was staring out
of the window. He was watching his wife. She was busily engaged in hammering
a FOR SALE sign into the lawn at the front of their house.

It is hard to express what that movie did to me, as it seared its way into my
consciousness. I was still trying to understand what the diagnosis might mean for
my life, to come to terms with what was happening to me. I yearned desperately
for something—some evidence, some information about research, some positive
example of a person living productively with M.S.—that would diminish the terror and give me a reason for hope. But, in large measure I lost my capacity for
hope that night—not entirely, nor permanently, but for many months to come. I
had been shown a detailed blueprint of the future, provided with a concrete and
vivid illustration of what lay in store for me. The process had already begun. The
only question that now remained in my mind was how rapid my destruction
would be.

I don't know what effect the movie had on my husband. We never spoke about it. Not on the way home in the car, nor in the days and weeks that followed. Two years later, at the time of our divorce, I wondered briefly if he (like me) had never been able to put it out of his mind completely. For months after seeing the film, whenever I tripped or dropped something, I thought of Joe.

As I reflect back on the impact of the diagnosis, I am forcefully reminded of the power of words and images to shape reality. The magazine story, the photographs, the film, the words of the physician (what he did and did not say), all influenced my understanding of what multiple sclerosis meant for my life. There is no doubt that the reality of my illness in the early days would have been other than it was if the initial "message" had been portrayed differently.

As it was, I spent the first few months after my diagnosis consumed with unrealistic and unnecessary fears. When I went to sleep at night, I was terrified that I might wake the next morning to find that my limbs would no longer move. I interpreted each and every insignificant muscle twitch as a portent of disaster. Every sensation—pins and needles, numbness, cold, cramp—suggested to me the beginnings of abnormal and permanent sensory loss.

Diagnoses, especially those that relate to serious illness, mean much more to patients than simply the identification of a particular disease state. Diagnoses are permeated with cultural and personal meaning. The dread diseases—cancer, heart disease, AIDS, multiple sclerosis—carry with them a particularly powerful symbolic significance. In living an illness, one is forced not only to deal with physical symptoms (numbness, weakness, pain, and so forth) but to wrestle with the question "What do these symptoms mean for ME, now and in the future?" In the case of incurable illness, this existential question is both urgent and profoundly disturbing. If one has a progressive disease, it is a question that must be addressed again and again.

In addition, one is forced to deal with the meaning that diagnosis has for *others*. Though multiple sclerosis does not carry the stigma of diseases such as AIDS and cancer, from the moment I was diagnosed people treated me differently. Even though I had no overt physical signs or symptoms, I was encouraged to "take it easy," to relinquish projects, to cut down on activities, to circumscribe my goals. The problem with this response from others, of course, is that it can become a self-fulfilling prophecy. I have met many M.S. patients who were persuaded that the diagnosis *in and of itself* required them to give up activities they enjoyed, to relinquish projects to which they were committed, and to make immediate and unnecessary revisions in their life plans.

I would probably have been similarly persuaded, except that I had no choice in the matter. Since my husband was a student, we were dependent upon my income. Even though I doubted I would be able to continue for long, I could not immediately give up my job. Having to go to work each day proved to be a blessing in disguise. It showed me, in a concrete way, that my life was not necessarily over.

Multiple sclerosis is a disease which is extremely variable, both in its course and in the manner in which the symptoms manifest themselves. As one neurologist put it succinctly, "M.S. is sort of like cancer—some kinds are not so bad, other kinds are awful." The disease most often strikes in early adult life (average age of onset is about thirty, with more women affected than men). Since it involves multiple lesions scattered throughout the central nervous system, symptoms are varied and may include motor weakness (most often in one or both legs but sometimes in arms and face), spasticity, incoordination, tremor, paralysis of the lower extremities, loss of balance, speech disorder, sensory changes such as numbness and tingling, visual disturbances (blurred or double vision), loss of bowel and bladder control, sexual problems, and a generalized lack of energy which manifests itself as chronic and easy fatiguability (Scheinberg 1983, 35–43). Clinically, multiple sclerosis may be categorized as a disease of the exacerbating-remitting type, in which discrete attacks of limited duration are followed by periods of recovery (although recovery may be incomplete, leaving some residual disability), or of the chronic progressive type, in which there is a steady accumulation of neurological deficit without remission. Chronic progressive multiple sclerosis usually evolves from exacerbating-remitting disease after a number of attacks, although approximately ten percent of patients have the chronic progressive form from the start (Weiner 1987, 442–444).

Since it is unclear what precipitates attacks, and because the course of the disease is unpredictable, uncertainty beleaguers the M.S. patient from the outset. This uncertainty not only relates to the prognosis but also involves treatment decisions. With exacerbating-remitting disease, there is some question as to whether the various treatment options bring about remissions, or whether recovery would have occurred with no intervention. With chronic progressive disease all modes of therapy remain controversial. The one thing about which all the experts agree is that there is no known cure.

Every M.S. patient has a different story to tell. The bewildering array of possible symptoms, together with the extreme variability in the severity and course of the disease, makes it difficult to talk about a "typical" course of multiple sclerosis. My own experience of the illness began with the loss of vision in my right eye, a symptom which lasted for several months and then abated. For a few weeks during that time, the vision in my left eye also became blurred and I lived with the quite terrifying prospect that I might become blind. In order to gain some control over my situation I went to the Lighthouse for the Blind and borrowed a book on braille. I managed to learn to read the dots of the braille alphabet but I never did develop enough feeling in my fingers to be able to interpret the raised letters. Gradually my vision returned to normal and, even though a recurring optic neuritis periodically robs me of sight in one or the other eye, I remain profoundly grateful for the ability to see. That short period when I could not drive, read a book, write a letter, or see clearly the faces of the people around me was without doubt one of the most frightening times of my life.

Over the ensuing months and years there were other attacks with different effects. That was the nature of my disease. Attack and then remission, attack and remission. Sometimes the remission was only partial and I was left with a new or increased disability.

The illness manifested itself in an astonishing variety of ways. I would experience a sudden weakness in one or more of my limbs, making it impossible to climb stairs (except on my hands and knees) or to walk more than a hundred yards without stopping to rest. One foot would begin to drag so that I tripped at every other step.

Once my hearing became so acute I could not bear to eat in a restaurant where every knife and fork seemed to screech against each china plate and the sound was multiplied a thousand times. I could not stand the noise of the typewriter, so I had to wear earmuffs in the office—the kind airplane mechanics wear to protect them from the noise of thundering jets.

Another time I lost the feeling in my leg. It was as if part of my leg had been injected with novocaine or had permanently "gone to sleep." I tried to massage it back to life, and soaked it in hot water, hoping magically to relieve the numbness. It didn't work. But I had to try something—anything—or be overcome with helplessness. Fortunately, that attack was short. I never could get accustomed to the sense of detachment, the feeling that the limb no longer belonged to me.

Still another attack affected my balance, causing me to stagger and weave like a drunken sailor. I hit walls, doorways, people—anything that got in my way. Judging by the disapproving glances I received in the grocery store, many onlookers assumed I was inebriated. That infuriated me, of course, and it made me very self-conscious. But I never said anything. What was there to say? I considered wearing a medical identification bracelet in case I was stopped for a traffic violation and asked to walk in a straight line.

Just when I thought I had experienced every possible symptom, my bladder refused to empty. I had almost perfected the technique for self-catheterization when bladder function reverted to normal.

One effect of my illness was constant from the very beginning. Fatigue. Every M.S. patient experiences debilitating, draining, bone-wearying exhaustion. This tiredness is unlike anything that one feels when one is healthy. Fatigue in M.S. (even for patients who have no overt signs of disability) means being able to walk into the grocery store in a normal fashion but being quite unable to walk out after going up and down one or two aisles. Exhaustion means sitting in a chair and being literally unable to move (to cross one's legs, to adjust the position of one's arm), or lying on the bed and being incapable of turning over, because it takes too much energy to do so. Fatigue is one of the most common and misunderstood symptoms of multiple sclerosis. It is invisible. Consequently, many M.S. patients who have no overt signs of their illness complain that they are berated for their lack of energy. They are accused of laziness, of using their illness as an excuse to get out of doing things, of being unreasonable in requesting time to rest, and so forth.

The acute attacks typically lasted for several weeks at a time. Occasionally they dragged on for a couple of months or more. I learned that the heat of summer (or hot water in the bathtub) made symptoms worse. Treatment consisted of the administration of steroids, either intravenously (which at the outset required hospitalization) or orally. I didn't like the effect of steroids. My body would become bloated, my face moon shaped. And I dreaded the IVs. My small veins were hard to find, requiring numerous, painful needle sticks. (Once when I had the IV administered at home by a professional nurse, she used more than fifty disposable needles in a ten-day period. Even when she got the IV started, the vein would collapse in a matter of hours and we would have to begin the process all over again.) But I did go into remission following treatment (not always immediately, but eventually). And, as important, treatment meant that I was doing something, that I had some control over what was happening.

I have focused on the periods of attack in order to give some sense of what it can be like to have multiple sclerosis. Yet (aside from the initial months of terror following my diagnosis) for many years my illness was the background rather than the foreground of my life. I could never totally disregard it, of course—the uncertainty about when the next attack might occur was always at the fringes of my consciousness—but, during the exacerbating-remitting phase of my illness, there were lengthy periods of remission during which I lived a relatively normal life. I continued to work full-time at my job as assistant to the executive vice president of a private university—albeit grudgingly giving up some other things that were important to me in order to compensate for fatigue. I completed part-time studies on an undergraduate degree. I often pushed myself to the limit and then had to pay the price of total exhaustion. But I was lucky. The things I most wanted to do did not require great physical exertion. Apart from my work, my passions were reading and listening to music. Things would have been different, of course, if I had wanted desperately to play tennis or if (like a physical education teacher I know) my job had required coordination and strength.

There were some particularly bad times, aside from the periods of attack. Less than two years after my diagnosis, my husband and I divorced. For me there was an added dimension to the pain and anguish of failure. For the first time I wondered if I would be able to manage on my own. The fear that I might become disabled intensified my anxiety about the future. I had always been very independent. I had supported myself since leaving school, had journeyed alone in my early twenties from my home in England to take a job as an executive secretary with an American oil company in North Africa. I had always believed that I could look after myself, that I had myself to depend on. When my marriage fell apart, along with my body, I lost that sense of confidence. That was one of the darker periods of my life.

But there were moments of great joy too. I remarried, spent a year in South Africa, and then returned to live in the States and began full-time graduate studies. In spite of a neurologist's prediction that I could not do it because I have M.S., I completed my doctorate in philosophy and began a new career as a teacher. Having M.S. did make it more difficult. Debilitating fatigue was my constant companion. And my illness robbed me of career opportunities. By the time I completed my academic studies I was physically able to teach only part-time rather than full-time. (Even in this I was fortunate: I had a long-standing relationship with the university where I teach; I would have had great difficulty obtaining employment elsewhere given my medical history.) However, my illness did not prevent me from having a meaningful life. My most important goal was to retain my independence, and, in large measure, that I was able to do.

About three years ago the pattern of my disease changed. There were no more acute attacks, but no remissions either. Rather, there began a slow but relentless, gradual progression of disability, in the course of which I have (among other things) permanently lost the full use of my legs, a good deal of upper body strength, my sense of balance, and normal voluntary control of my bowels and bladder. Over time I exchanged a cane for crutches, crutches for a walker, and—more recently—I relinquished the walker and began to use a battery operated scooter for mobility. Since the muscles that keep me upright have continued to weaken, I wear a back brace to give me some stability.

All treatment options for the chronic progressive form of M.S. are controversial. To have this illness is to confront firsthand the vast uncertainty of medical knowledge. But there is an enormous pressure on both the patient and doctor to do something, to intervene, to exercise some control. There must, after all, be something that can be done.

As my body visibly weakened, I began chemotherapy. I knew, of course, about its toxic side effects. I was aware that it increased my risk of cancer. I recognized that there was also no hope at all that it would cure my disease—only the possibility that it might slow down the rate of progression. I was to have monthly infusions with the prospect of continuing for a period of up to two years. The treatment was worse than the illness. Nausea, vomiting, and prostrating weakness made life miserable for two weeks out of every four. After three months, I discontinued therapy. The neurologist noted in his chart: "She does not want to do any more Cytoxan treatments unless or until she gets to the point where she cannot stand at all." *Unless or until.* There's the rub.

My progression has been marked by a series of seemingly mundane losses. I can no longer climb stairs, get up from a chair which does not have arms, turn over and get out of a king-sized bed, go through my back door into the garden, drive an automobile which does not have hand controls, get in or out of a bathtub which does not have grab bars, or carry a cup of coffee from the kitchen to the den.

I am, however, able to continue teaching and writing (as well as a host of other things which make my life eminently worth living). This is largely due to the unwavering support of my husband, who—besides bringing joy into my life and propping up my sometimes flagging resolve—cheerfully vacuums carpets, cleans floors, washes clothes, and studiously disregards the chaos occasioned by my total neglect of household chores. And to the help of my colleagues who rearrange their teaching schedules to suit my needs. I am also fortunate to have the economic resources to provide the means to compensate for my increasing loss of function—my electric scooter, my wheelchair, my handicapped-equipped van with hand controls, the ramp into my house to allow access, and so forth—otherwise I would surely be imprisoned by my body.

And I am blessed with a sense of humor, without which, I fear, my continuing losses might seem unbearable.

The answer to the question "What is it like to have multiple sclerosis?" is, however, only partially revealed in the description of its symptoms and the detailing of its course. For multiple sclerosis, like every other illness, is experienced not just as the breakdown of the body but as the disruption of the life that is lived in that body. Given the nature of the disorder, this life disruption manifests itself in different ways at different times. But since the disorder is chronic, the disruption is ongoing: even in periods of total remission, the M.S. patient lives with the disquieting knowledge that the disease is only temporarily quiescent. To live with multiple sclerosis is to experience a global sense of disorder—a disorder which incorporates a changed relation with one's body, a transformation in the surrounding world, a threat to the self, and a change in one's relation to others.

When we are healthy, we take our bodies very much for granted. For the most part, we speak, hear, and move unthinkingly as we go about our business, paying little attention to our physical capacities. Illness destroys this taken-for-grantedness. From the moment of diagnosis, I felt differently toward my body. In the first place, what was happening to IT was, more importantly, happening to ME. Whatever was going on in the deep recesses of my central nervous system (albeit incomprehensible, unfelt, unseen, unstoppable) threatened totally to disrupt my life. My body could no longer be trusted. Nor could it be ignored. I needed to be on my guard, to watch and listen to my body's rhythms, its sensations, its movements.

During acute episodes of illness, my body further intruded itself into my consciousness. Numbness called attention to my leg, weakness forced me to concentrate on the manner in which I picked up my foot, inserting a catheter into my bladder several times a day demanded that I focus explicitly on my incapacity to urinate. Rather than being that which was routinely overlooked, my malfunctioning body insistently and overtly reminded me of its presence.

Now that I am permanently disabled, this forced attention to body is ongoing. Although I do not brood about my illness, I must—as a matter of course—constantly take my body into account. It is the precondition of my plans and projects. Not only do I need to consider such things as fatigue and weakness, but I must constantly be aware of the limitations imposed by loss of mobility. For example, a routine invitation to someone's house, to the theater, to a professional meeting (or a trip to the grocery store, the post office, the shopping mall) requires that I first make inquiries as to whether or not I can get into the building (are there curb cuts, ramps, adequate parking, elevators). When I go on a trip, I must make arrangements for special accommodations (a bathroom with grab bars and wheelchair access), reserve particular seating on the airplane (close to the door, next to the aisle, within reach of the restroom), and so forth.

In addition, the effortful nature of movement requires that I pay explicit attention to my *dis*abilities so that I can better compensate for them. When sitting on the sofa I must, for example, manually position my legs if I am to push myself successfully into a standing position. Once upright, I must lock my knees if I am not immediately to fall back down again. While (in the course of time) I learn to carry out such compensatory movements almost unthinkingly, I am aware of my body's presence in the very act of performing them.

In the normal course of events we take for granted the effortless nature of movement. We do not marvel at the fluidity of motion, muscle strength, coordination, or balance, any more than we wonder at our ability to see or hear. Now that my muscles are weak and my movements uncoordinated, I perceive natural motion to be an extraordinary event. I catch myself watching students running across the campus, or colleagues taking the stairs two at a time, and I am amazed at the ease with which they manage it. Try as I might, I can no longer recall how it was to move like that.

Increasingly, my body also announces itself through the experience of absence. Limbs which will not move in accordance with one's wishes appear not only inert, lifeless, objectlike, but as no longer one's own. When I sit on the bed and try to lift my legs, I note to myself that *these* legs (not *my* legs) remain still. It is as if I am watching someone trying to move the legs. Earlier in my illness when I experienced a prolonged numbness in a limb, I felt as if that part of the limb were "dead." Now I have no numbness. I can still feel my legs. But I cannot move them in the most ordinary, mundane ways. This absolute impotence to control them causes me to feel detached from them and they from me.

Loss of mobility (be it prolonged or temporary) transforms the character of surrounding space. In the first place, what was formerly regarded as "near" is now experienced as "far." When I could walk, the distance from my office to the classroom (about 30 yards) was unremarkable. As my mobility decreased, the classroom appeared "near" to the office on the way to the lecture, but "far" from it on the return journey. Now, if I were to be without my motorized scooter, the distance to traverse would be immense—beyond attainable reach. The answer to the question "Is it too far?" no longer bears any relation to objective measurement of distance. It depends, rather, on what is *between* "here" and "there." Are there obstacles that prevent the use of my scooter? Is the terrain suitable for a wheelchair? (It may also depend upon my level of fatigue. In the morning I can—albeit with some difficulty—get from my bedroom to the den using my walker for support. By evening the distance is unbridgeable without my scooter.)

With loss of motility physical space assumes a restrictive character. Slopes may be too steep to climb, sidewalks too uneven to walk on, doorways too narrow to navigate with a wheelchair. Consequently, people with disabilities necessarily come to view the world through the medium of their damaged bodies. I well remember, for instance, that my first impression of the Lincoln Memorial was not one of awe at its architectural beauty but, rather, dismay at the number of steps to be climbed. It is interesting to note that friends and colleagues who regularly accompany me likewise come to view the world through the lens of *my* body; they routinely look for curb cuts, note access (or lack thereof) to buildings, automatically move furniture and other obstacles out of my path.

Until recently all of our architecture, every avenue of public access, was designed for people with working legs. This means that even when I am able to get into a building, I often have no choice but to do so by using the back entrance. I routinely make my way to conference rooms or restaurant facilities by means of a freight elevator, or sit in the stall of a public restroom with the door open (because the stall is not long enough to accommodate my scooter or wheelchair). I have visited many of the kitchens and laundry rooms in major hotels en route to otherwise inaccessible meeting places.

Obviously, the Americans with Disabilities Act (if properly enforced) will do much to open up public space. I remember a totally frustrating evening at a recent conference in Memphis when a colleague and I wanted only to walk a very short distance to a nearby restaurant. We were absolutely unable to get more than a block from the hotel *in any direction.* There were no curb cuts which would enable me to ride my scooter off one sidewalk and on to another. The accessibility of the restaurant itself was not an issue. I couldn't get to it. I could have taken a cab, of course, but the necessity for doing so illustrates the transformation in the character of surrounding space which occurs with loss of mobility. (In addition, taking a cab would have necessitated the dismantling of my scooter, considerable difficulty getting in and out of the back seat of the automobile, a special request to sit in the front, and so forth.)

Loss of equilibrium further alters the character of surrounding space. In the taken-for-grantedness of everyday life, the surrounding world presents a stable, nonthreatening environment. We stride down the corridor or across the parking lot, confident not only that our legs will function but that our senses will provide us with the necessary information to negotiate obstacles. We are oriented toward the world and the objects in it. To lose one's sense of balance is to become powerfully disoriented within the world. In the first place, it is to never know for certain that one can maintain one's position in space. I may be standing and suddenly, inexplicably, fall backward or pitch forward. I may intend to get out of a chair but, on pushing myself up, immediately fall back down again. Flat surfaces provide no more stability than uneven ones. Being "unbalanced" or "off balance" is to be vulnerable within the world. Before I used the walker or wheelchair my unsteady gait invariably caused me to bump into objects rather than going around them. It was simply a fact of life that I had permanent bruises on my shoulders from hitting doorways as I lurched through them.

Even open space is experienced as potentially threatening. Objects at least provide support. One way to negotiate space is to hold on to furniture or to touch walls. Open spaces can be frightening for those of us who have poor balance. (Perhaps an analogy will serve to give insight into this experience. Do you remember learning to ice skate—standing at the edge of the rink, faced with a seemingly immense expanse of ice and knowing there was nothing to hold on to once you let go of the barrier? And knowing also that you had almost no control of your legs once you ventured out onto the ice?)

A recent experience forcefully reminded me of the disconcerting character of open space. I was crossing the plaza outside the university library when my scooter stopped dead in its tracks. I was surrounded by a sea of concrete embedded with decorative pebbles, marooned in the middle of a flat, completely open area with no trees, no lampposts, no benches anywhere within reach. I did not have my crutches. There was no one in sight. The nearest "object" was the building, but it was impossible to reach it on my own two feet with nothing to support me. Nor could I easily crawl the distance, given the hard uneven surface of pebbled cement. And I was incapable of getting to my van (which contained a telephone and my crutches) since it was parked several hundred yards away at the bottom of a flight of steps. The space of the plaza, which a moment before had been bright, sunny, inviting, now suddenly appeared ominous. And in an instant, I recognized—in a new and chilling way—the magnitude of my limitations.

There is one further disruption of surrounding space which is a part of my experience of multiple sclerosis. With loss of function such everyday items as utensils, furniture, articles of clothing, and so forth have become problematic, requiring my unaccustomed attention. For example, swinging doors present a challenge to be negotiated with difficulty from my scooter or with my crutches; stairs are to be avoided or circumvented; a deep sofa is no longer an inviting resting place but rather one that is to be shunned (if I sit in it I cannot get up); to put panty hose on recalcitrant legs requires the assistance of a contraption that looks somewhat akin to a double taco holder with straps. Prior to my disability, when such objects were encountered they were barely noticed, if at all. Now that my body is incapacitated, I must explicitly attend to them.

In addition to the changed relation with body and the disruption of the surrounding world, serious illness is experienced as a profound threat to the self. From the very beginning I sensed that my illness represented a fundamental loss of wholeness—a loss of wholeness which related not simply to my physical state but, more importantly, to my personhood. That is, I felt my self diminished along with my body. Our sense of who we are is intimately related to the roles we occupy, professional and personal (wife, lover, secretary, woman, student), and to the goals and aspirations that we hold dear. Chronic, progressive, disabling disease necessarily disrupted (or threatened to disrupt) my every role in ways that, at the outset, seemed to me to reduce my worth as a person. Moreover, the uncertainty of the prognosis transformed my goals and aspirations into foolishness. This sense of diminishment was accompanied by a sense of guilt. I didn't have enough energy to do the household chores, I found it difficult to keep up with social activities, I needed extra time off from work, there were days when I had to ask others for help in the most menial of tasks. I realized that this was something over which I had no control. But still, in my heart of hearts, I felt in a myriad of ways that I was failing to do as I ought.

My divorce ratified this sense of failure. In retrospect I know, of course, that my marriage did not fail solely because of my illness (although it is an unhappy fact that many marriages do not survive the onslaught of M.S.). My illness was, if anything, simply the proverbial "straw that broke the camel's back." But, at the time, this particular failure increased my sense that what was happening to my body was directly related to my worth as a person.

Self-esteem is the easiest thing to lose with multiple sclerosis. And it may be the hardest to regain. This is, perhaps, particularly the case if motor function is disturbed. In this event, not only are roles disrupted in light of one's *disabilities*, but changes in movement patterns produce a body image which is overwhelmingly negative. This is a culture which places great value on physical fitness, sexuality, and youth. The person who staggers, wears a brace, uses crutches or a cane is far from the ideal. No matter how much one tries not to "buy into" this cultural imperative, the negative response of others is hard to ignore.

The loss of self-esteem is particularly profound with the loss of upright posture. Upright posture is directly related to autonomy. Just as an infant's sense of autonomy and independence is increased with the ability to stand upright and venture into the world unaided, so there is a corresponding loss of autonomy which accompanies the loss of uprightness. Not only does loss of upright posture engender feelings of helplessness and dependency in oneself, it also causes others to treat one as dependent. Whenever I am in my wheelchair, for instance, strangers tend to address themselves to my husband and refer to me in the third person.

"Where would SHE like to go?" "What would SHE like to drink?" At airports when we roll up to the security barrier, the attendant invariably asks "Can SHE walk at all?" We now have a standard response. My husband says, "No, but SHE *can* talk!"

This response from others is tempered somewhat when I am in my motorized scooter. However, I am still often treated in a condescending manner, as if I am a child. On almost every occasion when I go into a store, a customer or store clerk will make the following type of comment: "Oh, I wish *I* had one of those scooters. That looks like such fun!" I know they mean well. I understand that. And I know, too, that they have not the foggiest idea of what it can be like to lose the ability to walk. So, most of the time I smile politely (like a child) and try to ignore their condescension.

A sense of humor helps. One day, after watching me use the lift to get into my handicapped van, a woman walked up to the open car window on the passenger side and said to my mother, "Oh, SHE drives, does she?" My mother, slightly bemused by this inquiry, asked her to repeat herself. The woman looked straight at me, then turned to my mother and responded, "I see SHE drives, does she?" When I recounted this story to my husband he suggested my response should have been, "I have to go now. I'm late for my ballet lessons!"

Studies have shown that the views of the non-disabled toward persons with disabilities are overwhelmingly negative in this culture. This is particularly the case with respect to attitudes toward the disabled woman. Indeed, one disabled woman reports that whenever she and her husband are shopping and he is pushing her wheelchair, people come up to them and say to him, "You must be a saint"—the implication being that she is a burden and he is either saintly or a loser (Asch and Fine 1988). While this has not happened to me personally, people have remarked to me, "How *lucky* you are to have your husband." This is uttered not as a reflection regarding my husband's character but as a not-so-oblique reference to my disability—the perception being that, since I am disabled, I am a burden and that my relationship with my husband is solely one of dependence.

This perception on the part of others is particularly hurtful because it never fails to awaken one of my greatest fears—that, for all my good points, I am fast becoming a bother to those who love me. Progressive physical disability necessarily alters the dynamics of relationships, upsets the easy balance of give and take which is so important in the context of a shared life together. As I can do less, my husband, Dee, must do more. As my body inexorably weakens, it intrudes itself increasingly into our daily activities. I cannot help but wonder if a point will come when Dee will begin to resent the magnitude of this intrusion. For the past seventeen years he has been my greatest ally, reaffirming me in my sexuality, championing my efforts to retain some measure of independence, keeping me whole. We began our marriage vowing that together we would face the ongoing challenge of multiple sclerosis. Yet, I suspect neither one of us really understood how exacting the challenge would be.

In his research with people with disabilities, and in respect to his own personal experience of paraplegia, Robert Murphy has noted that the sense of diminishment experienced in disability is almost inevitably accompanied by a sense of shame. He recalls the following instance:

> I once suggested to a housebound elderly woman that she should use a walker for going outside. "I would never do that," she replied. "I'd be ashamed to be seen." "It's not your fault you have arthritis," I argued. I added that I used a walker, and I wasn't ashamed—this was untrue, of course, and I knew it. (Murphy 1987, 92)

Murphy goes on to note that this sense of shame is not rational; rather, it reflects the disabled person's subjective feelings of damage and diminished self-worth (feelings which are exacerbated by the negative response of others).

I, too, am ashamed of my disability. The feelings of shame have been most intense whenever I have had to adopt a new kind of mechanical aid to assist me in getting around (first the cane, then the crutches, then the walker, then the wheelchair and scooter). Most recently, I recall my anxiety that my students would think less of me if I came into the classroom on a scooter. So, for one whole semester, I rode the scooter down the hall, parked it *outside* the classroom, and lurched from the door to the podium on my own two feet! This was ridiculous, of course. I should have known better. Now that I routinely use the scooter and am familiar with the students' reaction (after the first day or two they simply accept my disability as a matter of course), I no longer worry. At least not in that now familiar situation—but I still feel self-conscious in the presence of strangers.

There is one bodily disorder associated with M.S. that causes particular shame. The loss of bowel and bladder control is much more than simply a mechanical or neurological dysfunction. Incontinence reduces an adult to the status of helpless infant. One is no longer master of even the most basic of bodily functions. So great is the threat of public humiliation that many afflicted patients simply choose to withdraw from society rather than risk embarrassment. Although I have, in time, become accustomed to most of my disabilities, I cannot view the loss of bowel and bladder control dispassionately. It is impossible to separate my self from my body in such a way that I do not feel, in some sense, violated on those occasions when I soil myself.

I have been asked whether I am angry that I have M.S. I suppose I am. But my anger is directed not so much at the "fact" of my being afflicted with multiple sclerosis as it is at the concrete manifestations of that illness in my everyday life. At the time of my diagnosis, I was, of course, for a short time preoccupied with the question "Why me?" What had I done to deserve this fate? But then I asked another question: "Why *not* me?" And I found this to be strangely liberating. Why not me? No reason. And since there is no reason, I felt free to put the question aside and to go on from there. I didn't (and don't) feel victimized. Multiple sclerosis is an unlucky break, and I wish I didn't have it. But I don't hold anybody responsible.

This does not mean, however, that I do not get frustrated, irritated, and sometimes downright furious at my body's incompetence to do the most simple tasks. And, perhaps, my greatest indignation is directed at the behavior of others—the ones who park in no-parking areas, blocking my handicapped van so that I cannot put down the lift and get back into it; the people who march unthinkingly through entrances and exits allowing swinging doors to slam in my face as I roll up behind them on my scooter; the able-bodied who treat me as if my inability to walk is indicative of severe mental retardation; and the physician who told me sternly that fecal incontinence was nothing. "Others have much worse things to deal with," he said, "and they do just fine. Just go out and buy some disposable diapers—but you need always to be conscious of the smell."

The problem with this anger, which is part and parcel of the experience of disability, is that it cannot be easily expressed. As Murphy has noted so well:

> [W]hatever the source of the grievance, the disabled have limited ways of showing it. Quadriplegics cannot stalk off in high (or low) dudgeon, nor can they even use body language. To make matters worse, as the price for normal relations, they must comfort others about their condition. They cannot show fear, sorrow, depression, sexuality, or anger, for this disturbs the able-bodied. The unsound of limb are permitted only to laugh. The rest of the emotions, including anger and the expression of hostility, must be bottled up, repressed, and allowed to simmer or be released in the backstage area of the home. . . . As for the rest of the world, I must sustain their faith in their own immunity by looking resolutely cheery. Have a nice day! (Murphy 1987, 108)

On those occasions when I have presented a paper relating to the experience of disability, I have almost always been asked by a member of the audience to state explicitly those things that I find "good" about my situation. Is it "enabling" rather than "disabling"? Has the experience caused me to "grow" in certain ways? I was once quite taken aback by a moderator who made the following, quite serious remark; "You have talked," he said, "about the constriction of space, and so forth, but couldn't you look on your disability as an advantage? After all, you don't have to exercise any more."

I was puzzled by this response until I read Murphy's remarks. Now I think I understand it better. But sorry, folks! Harsh though the reality may be, there is nothing intrinsically good about chronic, progressive multiple sclerosis. Nothing.

This is not, however, to deny that my life has been profoundly affected in ways that are enriching. The focus of my work (a focus that has brought me undeniable satisfaction) would undoubtedly have been different if I had been healthy. Some of my achievements, such as getting my doctorate, have been doubly sweet in light of the challenge of increasing disability. I have, no doubt, a greater understanding of the troubles of others, and a clearer view of what is really important in my life. I have also formed deep and lasting friendships with people who have journeyed with me in my illness, providing inspiration and support along the way. And I have, on many occasions, been touched by the kindness of others. I do not take these things lightly. They make my life worth living. They do not, however, make me glad that I have M.S.

Perhaps the greatest challenge of all for the multiple sclerosis patient is to learn to live with ongoing and permanent uncertainty. From the moment of diagnosis the future assumes an inherently problematic character. One does not know when the next attack will occur, how severe it will be, how long it will last, what effects it will have, whether there will be residual or increasing disability, whether treatment will be effective, or what the long-term prognosis might be. Neither does one know, on a day-to-day basis, whether one will feel energetic or abnormally fatigued, vigorous or enfeebled.

This pervasive uncertainty plays havoc with the patient's life. What becomes questionable, of course, is whether or not one has (or will have) the ability to complete professional commitments, participate in social events, and successfully carry out family responsibilities in the immediate or long-term future. Furthermore, the uncertainty about the prognosis affects the ability to project toward future goals. Are such goals "realistic," or maybe simply "foolish," in the face of the concrete threat of a progressively disabling disease?

When I was diagnosed with M.S. I was totally unprepared for such global uncertainty. People like me got sick, went to a doctor, got a prescription, took the medication, and got better. It was as simple as that. I knew, of course, of "others" who had incurable diseases. But the uncertainty of medical science was largely an abstraction. I had, for myself at least, an almost unbounded confidence in the power of medicine to restore me to health. (I realize this expectation is, to a large extent, nonrational. Even now—with all the evidence that I have to the contrary—I still catch myself saying, "There must be something that can be done.")

Such global uncertainty can have a paralyzing effect. I felt that I had absolutely no control over my situation, that I was, so to speak, totally at the mercy of my malfunctioning body. Since I could make no accurate predictions about the future, long-term goals seemed largely irrelevant. I was also deeply afraid. The future was not only uncertain, it was profoundly threatening. Would I become severely disabled? If so, when? Would the present incapacity become a permanent one? Of all the possible future scenarios that I could imagine, not one was the one I would have chosen for myself.

For some months after my diagnosis I simply went through the motions of living a life. I went to work, I continued my part-time studies for my undergraduate degree, I did the things at home that I had always done. But I felt in my heart of hearts that it was all a charade. There seemed little point in working for future goals when the future itself had disappeared.

I am not sure exactly when it was that I began to reclaim my life. Nor what enabled me to do it. Perhaps it was my day-to-day experience of M.S. which proved in a concrete way that I would not become immediately disabled. Or perhaps it was simply because I found living in constant fear unbearable. I do know that at some point I made a conscious decision to foreshorten my vision, to take one day at a time instead of thinking about next month or next year. I developed short-term rather than long-term goals: instead of focusing on the attainment of an undergraduate degree, I directed my energy toward completing one course; rather than concerning myself with possible future promotions at work, I concentrated on making it through the current week. It was not easy to focus exclusively on the present. But, as much as possible, I refused to allow myself to dwell on the future.

In turning to the present, I learned also to direct my attention from imagined difficulties to concrete ones. Rather than preoccupying myself with the future implications of a new disorder or disability (such as weakening muscles), I focused exclusively on the immediate disruption of my everyday life (for example, being too weak to stand at the blackboard and write during a fifty-minute lecture). Identifying concrete difficulties permitted me to develop specific strategies to deal with them (for this particular problem I could, for instance, start using an overhead projector). This put me back in control and thereby diminished the sense of global uncertainty.

This does not mean, of course, that I was no longer afraid. Every new attack revived my anxieties about the future. Each time, I had to begin anew actively to constrain my imagination, to reign in the latent feelings of terror. This was hard work. Some days I was more successful than others.

Now that my disease is actively progressive, I must face this fear more often. While I have not allowed the M.S. to become the focal point of my life, I experience ever more frequent epiphanies of increasing disability. A trip to the dentist following a three-month absence reveals I can no longer lift my legs on to the reclining chair; home movies taken a couple of years ago show me upright, walking with a cane; a visit to an old friend's house forcefully reminds me of what I already know—that (unlike the last time I visited) I can no longer go up the steps to the front door.

There are other triggers. I am teaching a class in medical ethics and the text cites two (or is it three?) cases involving patients with "advanced M.S." My neurologist, in discussing the pros and cons of estrogen therapy to prevent osteoporosis, tells me that I do not need to worry about falling and breaking bones—because I will not be able to stand up. The headlines debate the physician-assisted suicide of a multiple sclerosis patient in Michigan. Confined to a wheelchair, she tells her audience that she is no longer "living." She is merely "existing" and "existing is not enough." I note to myself that she is (was) younger than I am.

These are the thoughts that come unbidden in the night to reawaken my deepest anxieties. There is no way for me to look them in the face and remain intact. I must push them back. Back into the recesses of my consciousness. It is an act of will. I must think only of now. Of this day. Of this moment. Of what I have. Of what I can do. Of what gives me joy. Please, let me think only of this. Sufficient unto the day is the evil thereof.

In truth there is much to think about: the book I have recently finished, the paper I am writing, the professional meetings I plan to attend, the lectures I must prepare, the tests I must grade, the research I want to begin, the letters I should write. And I must drive my mother to the library, remember to take something out of the freezer for dinner, plan for the weekend when friends are due to visit. In the light of day I have little time to contemplate the terrors of the night.

And in the hurly-burly of living I am, for the most part, less inclined to focus on the dark side of my illness. There is within me (unasked for, uncultivated) an irrepressible sense of play which notes the sheer absurdity of the pickle I'm in— and laughs! I cannot take myself too seriously. Many of the things that happen with this disordered body of mine are funny—as well as frustrating and irritating.

I recall a recent trip to California. I was attending a philosophy conference at Esalen Institute, a place well-known for its somewhat avant-garde approach to psychotherapy. One afternoon I was outside, leaning on my crutches, attempting to take a photograph of two of my colleagues. I lost my balance and sat down on the grass. Since I have no muscle strength in my legs, I am dead weight when I fall. It is impossible to pick me up. So I asked my friends to get my wheelchair so that I could pull myself into it. To ensure that the wheelchair was level on the grass, it was necessary to position it some distance from where I had fallen and to face it in the opposite direction. My friends held the back of the chair firmly to steady it, while I crawled slowly along the grass toward them. Suddenly, a man with a flute appeared on the scene. (He was obviously an Esalen participant, no doubt enrolled in one of the many psychotherapy seminars.) He was horrified. From where he stood it appeared as if my friends were not only not helping me but that they were turning the wheelchair away from me. "Can *I* help you at all?" he asked indignantly. "No, I'm fine thanks," I replied. The man with the flute stepped back. He looked at me on the ground; he pondered my friends holding the wheelchair as it faced in the wrong direction. Suddenly he had a flash of inspiration. "Oh, I SEE," he said knowingly. "You're going through your PROCESS!" Then he turned and disappeared into the bushes.

In a sense I suppose he was right. I've been "going through my process" for nineteen years now. I might as well just keep on going.

NOTE

1. I should note that this is not intended as a criticism of the work of the M.S. Society. It was simply the case that, at this particular meeting, the individual in charge made what I consider to be a grievous mistake in showing this movie.

REFERENCES

Asch, A., and Fine, M. 1988. "Introduction: Beyond Pedestals." In M. Fine and A. Asch, eds., *Women and Disabilities.* Philadelphia: Temple University Press. pp. 1–37.

Murphy, R. F. 1987. *The Body Silent.* New York: Henry Holt and Company.

Scheinberg, L. 1983. "Signs, Symptoms, and Course of Disease." In *Multiple Sclerosis: A Guide for Patients and Their Families.* New York: Raven Press. pp. 35–43.

Weiner, H. L. 1987. "COP 1 Therapy for Multiple Sclerosis," *New England Journal of Medicine* 317(7): 442–444.

❖ 2 ❖

THE EXCEPTIONAL FAMILY
Walking the Edge of Tragedy and Transformation

RUTHANNE L. CURRY

Prologue

In writing this story as the mother of a physically disabled child, I returned to the handwritten journals which bore witness to our lives of the past sixteen years. From these pages where I had initially tried to make sense of our pain, grief, and occasional triumph emerged recurring themes or threads of meaning. I have attempted in the following story to share these meanings, including excerpts from my own journals which seemed particularly illustrative. Reflecting upon earlier struggles and experiences has been a difficult process, but one which has offered further healing. While this experiential account represents my memory of our family's evolution as an exceptional family, the "story" is a continuing one.

Others, who have kindly shared their thoughts and impressions after reading my story, have suggested that I offer the reader an orientation to our family. We are a family of four: mother, father, older sister, and younger brother, Robbie, who is the child with the disability. While our roles as father-physician and mother-nurse practitioner have colored our experiences, it is our voice as an exceptional family which I wish the reader to hear.

Walking the Edge

THIS IS A STORY about an exceptional family—a family labeled as different because of the son's chronic disability. In many ways, they are ordinary. They go to work, attend school, eat dinner together, get colds, worry about money and their future. Yet always coloring their predictable survival tasks and concerns are the son's needs and society's expectations. People around them may want them to be particularly brave or carefully grateful, as if their "differentness" requires them to be more than just ordinary. To gain entrance or acceptance into the mainstream, they must carry their differentness well or risk being pitied. Few allow them their humanness. Those who do share their journey offer the richest resource.

The journey begins with two major conflicting forces: hope and sorrow. As in most families, the son's beginning was anticipated with much excitement. His unexpected premature birth exposed their vulnerability; they were no longer "normal." Saddened by a lost pregnancy and pummeled by fears of what was to come, the mother adopted a "Mother Bear" stance with the tiny baby. Her son became the first preemie to be breast-fed in the small rural hospital, nurturing both his survival and her hope that he would emerge intact.

> Twelve hours after birth, Robbie is deemed ready for visitors. Delivering prematurely somehow seemed to relegate our status to that of privileged third cousins rather than parents. I would finally be allowed to hold my child. His physician father would wait ten days for Robbie's first touch. Approaching the incubator alone, my hands stroked Robbie's fragile, utterly soft body. Amid wires, beeping equipment, and doubtful glances, I put Robbie to breast as I had my first child. Although smaller and weaker, he responded as she had. We would repeat this scene many times, our shared warmth reassuring us. We belonged together.

Other than prematurity, there were no visible or dramatic markers to identify the insidious damage which had occurred in the baby's brain. Hope continued to gently flourish as the now family of four entered the son's infancy. When the baby was six months of age, however, his inability to sit or roll over allowed the earlier fears surrounding his wholeness to return. Although the parents desperately wanted their child to be "normal," the baby's slow development shouted otherwise. Tentative questions to professionals were often met with comments meant to be helpful and reassuring. Finally, the toll of daily battle with an unknown enemy demanded action and the first of many "experts" entered their lives.

> After months of suppressing doubts about Robbie's development, I seek the opinion of a developmental psychologist. Now, all my rationalizations linking slow development with prematurity crumble before the psychologist's gentle but persistent words. Something, some disease or injury, shrouds Robbie's body as surely as my arms now cradle him. Future visions of children struggling with crutches or clouded intellects kaleidoscope with the reality of the warm baby against me. Worries of what is to come collide with terrible questions about what has happened to our son. Hours later sitting on my couch at home, I feel as though I might drown in the crashing pain. I did not know that our survival would de-

mand repeated encounters with this maelstrom. But this moment would hurt the most.

So the family began to weave their differentness into the everyday tasks of making a life. While other parents went to work or school, this mother took the baby to physical therapy or the ophthalmology clinic or a class for "at risk" babies. No one had spoken a diagnosis, leaving room for continued hope but also ambiguity. Just what were they dealing with anyway? Most of the time, the commitment to doing something minimizes their feelings of helplessness and brings some small progress. At other moments, the continued encounters jar them into realizing just how compromised their son is.

Each baby class brings more and more healthy babies who roll, crawl, babble, throw things. These incredible creatures are a half, a third Robbie's age. It's like being in the desert and watching someone else drink an incredibly cold drink. I want to shake these other mothers. Do they know how wonderful this all is? But I am too proud to admit my longing.

After several months of many therapy sessions and hearing others comment on their son's problems, the parents choose to begin an all-out assault on whatever process has laid claim to their child. As all successful wars begin with excellent intelligence reports, they turn to specialists in the large medical center in their community. They are ready for the facts.

How strange it feels to be in the role of "patient's mother." The waiting room of the large clinic is tense with families tired from filling out papers, consoling difficult children, and worrying about their impending visit. As I look around at all the children, I am struck by the terrible devastation. So many of them seem helpless and defenseless, as if they are casualties of some awful catastrophe. Is this how others see my child? I want to clutch our son and hide somewhere. Later, the words which have already reverberated in my head are pronounced by the neurologist: cerebral palsy. As he reviews the findings, a door slowly shuts. While there will be no miracle, neither will Robbie die soon. As we leave the clinic carrying our reprieved son, the ghost of Robbie-might-have-been begins to drift away.

While the parents have begun to live with ghosts, others in the family are lagging behind in the journey. The grandparents, seeing their own children's pain and energy depletion, want to help. As they are often separated by time and distance from the day-to-day survival which the parents must face, they are partially insulated from the struggle. They must find their own way to live with this different grandchild.

We have taken the children to visit Whit's parents, hoping for a change in our endless round of clinic appointments and therapy sessions. I sense that they are both excited and nervous about our coming. After all, their questions and understanding have been filtered through our interpretations of what others have told us. Although I want to be sensitive to their possible distress, we are in great need of comfort ourselves. As Whit's mother and I sit on the lakefront shore rocking slowly in the hammock with Robbie, I tentatively expose my hurt.

"It's as if someone has died," I tell her. I can feel her recoil. My words have been too honest.

"You just have to be strong," she replies. I wonder if I must be strong to protect her as well as my son.

Like many other families, this one is linked by the usual holiday dinners and birthday parties. These expected encounters promote repeated inoculation to Robbie's assets as well as his liabilities and allows the other, more distant family members to become comfortable with his slumping body posture or raking grasp. Some move more easily into his style, and offer the friendly acceptance the parents crave for him.

My mom and dad have come to Florida to enjoy their grandchildren and escape the cold. Mary K. is jumping with "Grandma" projects to do, and I am again glad to have some adult conversation. As I merge breakfast routine into getting Mary K. ready for preschool, Mom and Dad take Robbie. I glance over at the happy, ordinary sounds coming from our couch. My parents are tickling Robbie and blowing bubbles with total glee. The young baby, who is more likely to cry or fuss, is responding with giggling abandon. They have taught Robbie to laugh. How simple, but how needed.

Family members learn to savor these moments of happiness, tucking them into their collective memory to sustain them on other less sunny days. The roller coaster of hope and sorrow, physical exhaustion and encouragement continues to require balance reactions which they are learning to cultivate. Guilt, rage, fear, and frustration repeatedly threaten to suck them down into perpetual grief, but the son always seems to pull them back with his sheer commitment to be.

June 22nd—almost the longest day—how I feel that our lives seem to be composed of "long" days. How absurd that I should want to give up at times. My son is the one with the disability. I could walk away if I really wanted to, yet can he? Sometimes I just want to be with him without all the "should's" of doing therapy at home, clinic appointments, reinforcing appropriate behavior, nurturing, and dressing, while fighting off the guilt monster. I wonder what he really wants. He tries to tell me with cries or by tightening his body. I am so used to reading his nonverbal ways that I almost missed his first "real" talking. Today he called me "Ma" for the first time. After two and a half years, he can finally call me, acknowledge me as a person. While other children have been able to crawl after their parents, he has had to cry or fuss to seek us out. Now he has another way to engage us besides crying.

Language validates many of the ways in which the family see Robbie, an individual who seems to grasp quickly much of what occurs around and with him. While family members have bridged their relationship with him through touch, holding, smiling, carrying, and generally bringing the world to him, his verbal reciprocity now further reinforces their efforts to work with him. In contrast, daily encounters with less observant or informed individuals force the family to somewhat reluctantly share their impressions with strangers. Advocacy is not in their everyday vocabulary but soon becomes mandatory.

Lunch at McDonald's, a most American custom, is even more than just lunch with the kids. Robbie has finally taken to eating meat—McDonald's hamburgers. Even this is ironical after all the homemade baby food and other "healthy" concoctions I have created. He attacks the food in his usual less-than-precise style. At the adjoining table the children have obviously raised some questions to their now uncomfortable mother who starts muttering and casting us furtive glances. I can feel the anger starting to seep into my awareness. Although I am a nurse, I would seriously like to clobber this woman for telling her children "he is a victim" and "not to look." Do I owe her an explanation? Somehow, if I am to help my son see himself differently than this woman does, I must do something. I smile at the children and begin my awkward public relations attempts.

"It's o.k. to wonder what happened that he moves differently than you do. His brain was hurt around the time he was born, but he's not sick (I have learned some kids think they might "catch" it) and in many ways is just like you."

The kids now sense the floor is open to questions. When will he walk? Why does his eye look away? Will he die? I gulp. Am I ready for this? Scared or not, I have waded into this and best bumble some sort of finish. I hear myself explaining haltingly that we hope he will walk, that he will not die soon, and his eye seems different because those muscles are not working together. The kids, satisfied with those answers, return to their hamburgers. I look down at the crushed french fry in my hand.

Over the subsequent months and years, it is often the children who help the family find their way. Friends' children, occasional visiting cousins, and most of all the daughter, Mary K., often figure out how to live with Robbie. Five-year-old Mary K. and her friends pile their supplies around Robbie in the red wooden wagon and venture off in the make-believe "frontier" behind their house. Other toddlers play alongside him briefly and take his toys; Robbie learns to verbally try to stop them. The children of new acquaintances sometimes also provide a bridge to other parents.

My new neighbor Linda bikes by our backyard where Rob and I are "experiencing" the sandbox Whit has created. On the back of Linda's bike is her son, Tim, who is a few months younger than Rob. Linda is bubbly and friendly, calling out to us and introducing herself. We chat and at some point I feel I must explain Robbie's obvious differences from her son. Somehow, this part always feels like a test. Will my "orientation" to Robbie's difficulty honestly present his compromises without scaring people away? Linda responds with a mixture of interest and friendly concern. When she mentions that she plays tennis every week, I offer to have Tim stay with us while she plays. We are always looking for playmates. She agrees, but on the condition that I leave Rob with her for an equal amount of time. I am startled. Linda is the first friend to offer to brave Robbie alone.

Other mother-child pairs become part of the family's efforts to rescue their lives. Bike rides to the park, picnic lunches, and walks through neighborhoods relieve the isolation of nurturing a young child eighteen hours a day. Sharing everyday events and the boundless energy of other mothers' children allows the parents to see their son as more like other children than so singularly dissimilar. The family needs these friends and strangers-become-friends like they need food. Despite their need, the parents sense there are rules for this game of social integration. Most of the time they feel they should initiate contact, explaining the disability to newcomers and readily appreciating inclusion. Part of their consciousness is always censoring what they share lest they lose their "admission" to the ordinary world. They find an emotional closet in which to store their feelings. The closet is opened only with a few tested friends or in moments of reckless bravery.

When their son is three years old, the parents have the opportunity to experience a divergent world where disability is now the entering ticket. They leave familiar home territory and travel to Washington, D.C., living for five weeks in a college dormitory with thirty other parents and children growing up with disabilities. All these people have come together to offer their children as "practice subjects" for therapists learning new techniques to help their children.

Initially, I realize we are checking each other out, wondering about the children's problems, curious about adaptations others have found, and amazed that there could be so many of us. We are all like wounded geese, still flying on an altered course to assist our children. While our lives have never been the same since our children arrived, we have all survived. That in itself is a miracle. I am humbled by the commitment of these other parents and immensely relieved that

I am not alone. I am also aware that my troubles sometimes pale in comparison to what other parents are managing. Somehow known problems seem less overwhelming than scenarios I never imagined. It is our commonality of experience, however, which leads to new understanding.

One night, Celia, home economist by training and mother of blond, chipper Kristen, and I share a moment over chicken noodle soup prepared in the dorm kitchen. Celia has ventured into that gray land called "the future," wondering whether Kristen will be a "domestic ambulator"—someone who can walk around the house but not to the store. This has already proceeded beyond the bounds of the usual chats I have had back home but I hear a familiar thread of my own thoughts. Suddenly, Celia looks up at me.

"What if she can't cook for herself?" she asks.

I am not sure how to respond. Is she asking whether Kristen will be dependent on her or others? I know this song, except mine involves my son getting a job. I realize we may define our children by what matters to us rather than who they are. I hear myself offering Celia the idea that her tenacious, bright but stubborn daughter might become a lawyer and hire a housekeeper. Celia laughs with relief, partly because I have suggested a hopeful solution but more because we have been afraid together.

Five weeks of intensive therapy and spontaneous, close relationships with other "different" parents lead the family down new paths. Fifty therapists, thirty children and parents, and ten therapy faculty all blend into a stimulating "soup" of alternatives and energy. Until now, the parents have repeatedly struggled with a bipolar concept of their child; he would walk, talk, learn, socialize, and grow up, or he would be disabled. They actively resisted seeing his disability as part of who their son was because to do so seemed to be giving up. To be disabled also seemed to mean passivity, helplessness, victimization. Out of their experiences with these other parents and therapists emerges a fresh recognition of who their son might be, a person who happens to have severe movement problems. He also "happens" to have a wonderful smile, an intense will, and a bright mind. They are beginning to learn how to live with the enemy, but are still vigilant that the cerebral palsy be allowed few concessions.

Blond, hazel-eyed Robbie leans against the gigantic beach ball while the therapist attempts to reduce his marked stiffness. Near the end of the hour-long session, which he has tolerated with little crying today, the therapists rock him slowly onto his feet. He stands with their help, an almost casual awareness that he is both relaxed and upright at the same time. Another mother quickly snaps a polaroid picture, as I am so engrossed by the look in Robbie's eyes, I have forgotten the magnitude of this moment. The standing may be a window to other, more independent movement, but it is his expression of belonging in this body which I will remember.

The family's growth during the summer of therapy away from home facilitates new skills and social courage. After participating in a parent session focusing on education, the parents decide to merge their hope for a preschool experience for their son with their commitment to push local school board members toward offering an early education program. The school administration has deferred the family's inquiries to the elected members of the board, who must decide whether money will be spent to start an early education program. The parents contact the individual board members one by one and arrange to meet with them. Several are supportive of the concept of early education, while others apparently need help in understanding the problems and possible solutions.

Robbie and I are again on our way to meet Whit and school board member number three at the restaurant of his choice to discuss the lack of preschool opportunities. As we enter the restaurant, Mr. H. politely shakes our hands. Although he attempts to mask his surprise that we have included Robbie, I recognize the now familiar averted gaze and general uncomfortableness. I sense this will not be easy. After presenting our now well-rehearsed "talk" and reminding the board member of the intent of Public Law 94–142, we pause, waiting for him to respond. By now our food has arrived and Robbie has begun to awkwardly feed himself. I have ordered him a pancake, a food with which I knew he would have some success but produce limited mess.

Mr. H., nodding his head toward Robbie asks, "Why does your son need a program? I mean, he can feed himself." Because, I want to say, life should be more than eating pancakes.

While the parents continue to juggle their developing advocacy with their son's needs, their impatience grows. Their efforts at increasing their own awareness and knowledge about their son's disability repeatedly point toward early intervention. They are racing a developmental clock which is already several years late. An educational experience will also offer another way for their son to begin to learn how to live with his peers. The parents decide to explore other regular community preschools.

Tomorrow Robbie and I are to attend a private preschool. Through phone calls and luck, I have found the director of a community college program which trains special education aides and a preschool director willing to consider Robbie's attendance with one of these trainees. Tomorrow will be another "coming out"—of facing new people and new situations where the possibility exists for misunderstanding, comparison, and rejection. Yet, tomorrow is, more importantly, another opportunity for everyone to grow a little—Robbie, the teachers, the "normal" kids. Please let my determination help us see the possibilities.

The preschool experiment works. Again the children lead the way with their pragmatic curiousity and problem solving. Once they grasp the new child's limitations and abilities, they learn to move with him in a dance of give and take. Sometimes they run away and he cannot follow. Other times, they are more likely to play alongside him or laugh at his spontaneous participation. The parents are encouraged by their child's language explosion, his willingness to reach out toward other children, his evolving trust in others outside his own family. From the lack of a special education setting has emerged an early model for integration. The family will continue to seek other integrated school settings as Robbie grows older. If he is to have a life beyond therapy, clinic visits, and family protectiveness, he must learn to deal with the fears and questions of others now. They have figured out that school is a microcosm of society; learning is more than knowing one's letters and numbers.

As family members continue to move reluctantly into arenas they never envisioned, the problem of helping the son form an identity which both includes and goes beyond his disability impacts everything they do. Through their small advocacy efforts and contacts with professionals who deal with disabilities, they are now visible outside their circle of friends and neighbors. The system appears to see them as a compromised but marketable example.

Before running out the door to therapy, I grab the phone. One of the public school therapists whom I barely know wants to know if smiling, five-year-old Robbie might be the March of Dimes poster child. Immediate conflict starts to churn in my gut. I am torn between wanting to be a team player through doing a good deed for the community and a nagging sense that this somehow just does not feel right. I have learned to ask questions before "buying" anything.

"What does the March of Dimes use their money for?" I ask her. "Does any of it go for the treatment or programs many of the children need?"

She explains that the money is used for research to prevent prematurity, birth defects, and other health problems with which the children are born. I hear myself fumbling with an answer tinged with irritation and sadness.

"I'm sorry," I explain, "but I don't feel comfortable telling my son that he is doing this to prevent other children like him. We're trying to help him understand where he fits into a world that is often more confused than he is about his problems. I can't put him out there as something to "prevent." This poster thing also seems to use these kids to collect money, yet you tell me none of it goes toward addressing their problems now. That feels sort of dishonest."

I realize I have given away potential "celebrity" status for Robbie by declining their invitation. I have also risked being labeled an ungrateful parent. But I think I have been true to what I really want for him. Free lunches and pictures in the newspaper are not going to help him push his wheelchair into a community that sees him as something that should not have happened.

Ten years later, Robbie will choose to "walk" his wheelchair thirteen miles in the March of Dimes Walk-a-thon as part of his Boy Scout service project. There will still be no newspaper pictures, just quiet accomplishment in doing something for others. The journey between possible poster child and teenage contributor, however, will require the family to rework earlier struggles. "Anniversaries" often force open the closeted feelings and offer bittersweet opportunities for growth.

Just-turned six-year-old Robbie sits in a small child-sized chair, secured by a velcro strap and a homemade knee abductor. Many of his schoolmates surround him as he opens their carefully chosen presents. There are all sorts of books and bookmarks, for the children have observed Robbie's new mastery of reading. There is also a slate upon which Robbie can easily draw and a car which he can activate by just pushing down. I am appreciative of the children's and their parents' sensitivity to what might be an appropriate gift for Robbie with his limited mobility. We have had a fun day, playing with the children and helping Robbie participate in the games he has planned. As we clean away the cake crumbs and shredded paper, I am thankful for the friends who have helped make this a "typical" happy birthday. Although I smile as I remember Robbie directing me in the party peanut hunt, I feel another year of hoped-for progress needing readjustment. In many ways I keep losing him over and over—relinquishing the child that never was, letting the dreams, however unrealistic, slip away, reshaping my vision of what he might be. We have come so far, always trying compassionately and persistently to push and guide him toward his own life. Yet, I am forever wondering if we have held him too close, found the right therapy or education, given the most genuine parts of ourselves 29 hours a day. Sometimes it seems as if we want him too much. Sometimes I want for just one moment for the disability to let him be.

In their recurrent encounters with sadness, the family attempts to find some explanation or meaning. Having been figuratively struck by lightning, they realize the unfairness of life's events. Neither do they believe in a "grand plan" theory; no higher force has selected them or the child for martyrdom or punishment. Just as they will never know what biological process or medical oversight led to the son's problems, neither will they be able to foresee the future. What has happened is put aside; what will come is dealt with as a present-day here-and-now dilemma. They learn to slowly, repeatedly forgive themselves for possible past mistakes and current omissions.

I am alone in the library, writing in the journal which has long been my honest friend. As I write, I am aware that the guilt I sometimes feel is now only a vague reminder of a way of living that helped me cope for so many years with fear. When something terrible happens in your life, you either feel that "it finally got you" or you see the total absurdity of that fearful superstition. For so long I believed that if I followed the rules, gave my best, or did the "right" thing, I might accomplish something or at least escape some painful fate. Now I know that if there ever were any rules, they have been broken. What an incredible sense of freedom Robbie has given me.

As the family continues to grow alongside the child with the disability, they learn to rely upon a core of discovered beliefs. These sometimes painfully forged "truths" about themselves, the child, and the world in which he will someday live without them are woven into their daily lives. Often when they are exhausted from the physical and emotional demands of caring for the child, their frustration makes them ask the "why" and "where are we going" questions. There are, of course, the immediate, concrete goals for the child, such as learning to drink from a straw or to drive a new electric wheelchair. The once ultimate goal of walking, so symbolic of independence, is now fading, however. The family must again choose between despair and redefinition.

We have nervously assembled in the large community college auditorium for the Montessori end-of-the-year school play. Our daughter Mary K., several grandparents, friends, and therapists have all come to watch "Peter Pan," who will be played by a blond boy in a red wheelchair. Robbie's incredible memory and unselfconscious singing have landed him the lead. During the play, several lines are muffed, a mermaid trips on her tail, and Robbie's voice projects less than optimally. For the exhilarating "I'm Flying" scene, a creative costume designer has rigged a way for Robbie to fly across the stage. As I anxiously hope the harness will hold Robbie, a stage hand gives Robbie/Peter a big push. Robbie looks more like a suspended fish than a trapeze artist, but the imagery is there. Robbie, who may never walk, is flying. In many ways, he has also learned to fly with his spirit.

What the parents may want for their son and what they think he may want for himself frequently distill into intangibles. While they have become credible troubleshooters at integrating their son into his surroundings, they often return to their sense of underlying purpose to direct their actions and renew their efforts. Self-esteem, love, and the ability to be touched by the moments of life serve as the family's anchors.

We have just come back from another three weeks of intense therapy with our friend and therapy "expert" Chris. Going to work with Chris is like taking your child in for a major overhaul of ideas, approaches, and creative equipment. She, like many of the therapists who have listened, cared, and given their best, infuses us with energy and a "can do" attitude. Somehow she knows how to help us translate our dreams into what we need to do today without overwhelming us. Watching her touch Robbie involves seeing more than the obvious movements. She asks him with her hands to continually let go of his spasticity, to trust her to lead his body into subtle new sensations. In offering him a guided way to try something different, she validates who he is now and who he might become. I am aware that therapy is considerably more than creating possibility for movement. The intense relationship between the therapist and Robbie reflects many of the less visible experiences I want for him—to try and not quite master it but still count for who he is now. As I observe Chris and Robbie work together, I remember a line in "The Little Prince."

"It is only with the heart one can see rightly," the fox says to the Little Prince. "What is essential is invisible to the eye."

As other individuals care for and about the child, the parents' perceptions of their son are reinforced. Acceptance of his evident disability is more than a scientific diagnosis and evaluation of what he can or cannot do. To be able to hope for love for their child in the larger world outside their family, the family members need help in molding a loveable and loving individual. While the parents expend incredible energy, time, and interest in addressing the disability, they also learn to treat him more as a child than as a health problem. This requires vigilant awareness. While their son has many needs and limited abilities, their expectations are often directed by the behavior of their daughter. Her development serves as a compass for the uncharted course they travel with their son.

Vibrant, talkative Mary K. runs through the house collecting materials for her next drama production. Her more quiet friend Laura follows, pushing Robbie in his child-size wheelchair. Robbie is not too sure he wants to participate, but the girls coax him into giving it a chance. Lesson 241: If one wants to be included, one needs to be flexible. After the children's magic show in which Robbie produces a puppet rabbit from an old hat with Mary K.'s sly assistance, they decide to go swimming. Lesson 242: Disability or not, life moves quickly. As we later play in the pool, I remember that Mary K. will be leaving soon for four weeks of overnight camp. We will all miss her dearly. That feeling leads to another "lesson." Every child needs the opportunity to get away from her or his parents. In our family, I must fight to protect Mary K.'s right to move away from us. I must also find a way for Robbie to leave us.

Leaving the family's immediate circle of care and understanding does occur through school, through driving the wheelchair down the street, and eventually by going away to camp. Each separation arouses manageable fears which are amplified versions of what the parents experienced with their daughter. Will their son be physically safe? Will others acknowledge his abilities and allow him to try? Will he have fun? Can they trust him to find his way, however hard that may be? Some separations are more difficult than others.

As we kiss Robbie good night, my words of encouragement attempt to mask my concern. Tomorrow Robbie will face the first of many surgeries. For ten years he and the hours of therapy have kept the surgeons as mere observers. Although tempted to seek surgical "fixes" for Robbie's problems, I have chosen to trust the therapists more. Now we are forced to decide between possibly limiting future mobility and surgically transferring muscles, which may compromise what little function he has. I have always wanted options in his care and demanded participation. I am acutely aware though that our responsibility exacts a price. Robbie will have to live with the consequences of our decision. Will he blame us if things do not go well?

Hours later, as we wait for the surgery to be over, the crisis of an unknown outcome allows prior battles to resurface. I remember how it felt each time I explained my way into the newborn nursery years ago, wondering what had happened to my child in my absence. What if Robbie were to die now? For so long we have fought to find a way around, through, over, or in spite of the disability, so that the child in Robbie might have a chance. What if this is a gamble we should never have taken?

Other surgeries will provoke similar fears. While the disability requires the family to dance with it rather than attempt to control it, hospital settings often overlook much of what the family has mastered. Even in a health care environment, where physical compromises are everyday occurrences, patronization and underestimation appear. While the parents know there are few ways in which medicine may help their son, they hoped that their fellow health care professionals might see the individual in their child.

I arrive in the pediatric intensive care unit where Robbie has stayed after his third surgery. He will be moved today to the pediatric floor after a quiet night. The nurse who has cared for him has attempted to give him choices in his care and he seems relatively pain-free. As I remove the Walkman headset from his ears, the nurse comments on how he listened all night to his Bill Cosby tapes. Robbie has learned that humor is definitely one way to deal with this experience. Chuckling herself, the nurse remarks on how strange it was to hear Robbie laugh through the night. Her comments reveal how absent this place is of laughter. I wonder also if she thinks disabled people are incapable of having fun in other settings.

Several days later on the pediatric floor, Robbie and his older, but mentally younger roommate, Tom, are watching a television program together. A young, abrupt woman resident whips into the room, yanks the curtain closed and proceeds to do an invasive procedure on the roommate. Frightened, Tom begs her to stop.

Suddenly, immobile Robbie yells to the physician, "He doesn't understand what you are doing. You need to tell him or leave him alone."

The resident peers around the curtain, unsure as to who initiated this directive. Embarrassed by two teenagers, she is not sure how to proceed. She eventually examines the roommate but Robbie has managed to assert himself from a prone position.

As the teenager grows up, issues which have always been there assume new importance. While their son was young, the parents dealt with the uncertainty of his future through believing that they must somehow outlive him. Gradually they realize the impracticality and unhealthiness of this idea. Again they will have to trust him to deal with the outside world, just as he has negotiated other difficult situations. Their son will still need some "road maps" and occasional directions, but hopefully they have given him the essentials.

The almost empty college gym echoes with the voices of the basketball players Robbie has come to watch. One of the university sports information directors has invited him to observe practice, having learned of Robbie's obsession with sports and his budding interest in a sports information career.

Years ago, I once asked Robbie if there were things he wished he could do. He answered simply, "I'd like to be able to run—not walk, but RUN."

Today as I watch him intently follow the players' moves, I know he is attempting to run with them through his head. There will be the predictable real and psychological obstacles. Will he be able to attend college, live with other young adults, find a job? Will someone appreciate his strengths and see who he may continue to become?

He and the sports information director are now going over player statistic sheets and talking about the press coverage for tomorrow's game. I am just another observer of the practice session. And that is what it has all been about. . . .

❖ 3 ❖

CHRONIC ILLNESS AND THE
DYNAMICS OF HOPING

DAVID BARNARD

> The truth is that there can strictly speaking be no hope except when the
> temptation to despair exists. Hope is the act by which this temptation is
> actively or victoriously overcome.
>
> —GABRIEL MARCEL, *HOMO VIATOR*

> Fear of the future and flair for confronting it are complexly intertwined;
> I want to pick away at the threads, to explore the tangle.
>
> —LIONEL TIGER, *OPTIMISM: THE BIOLOGY OF HOPE*

WHEN HOPE IS spoken of in medical settings it almost always seems to be in an extreme situation. Someone is either facing terminal illness or death ("Let us convey the news so as not to remove all hope"), or has sustained a catastrophically disabling injury—a severed spinal cord, say, or massive burns ("We must keep him alive, despite his insistent demands to let him die, until his depression lifts and hope returns"). These concerns are real, and attention to hope is certainly a critical part of the care of people in such circumstances. However, there is another very large realm of experience where hope and the dynamics of hoping are equally at home, but a realm which is less often mentioned as a context for hope: the everyday world of the chronically ill and disabled.

The relative lack of attention to chronic illness, disability, and hope is especially remarkable because chronic illness and disability disclose the very aspect of human existence that gives birth to hope, namely, that human beings are poised on the boundary between finitude and transcendence. Ernest Becker, albeit in somewhat overheated prose, describes this boundary as the "existential paradox":

Man has a symbolic identity that brings him sharply out of nature. He is a symbolic self, a creature with a name, a life history. He is a creator with a mind that soars out to speculate about atoms and infinity, who can place himself imaginatively at a point in space and contemplate bemusedly his own planet. . . . Yet at the same time . . . man is a worm and food for worms. . . . Man is literally split in two: he has an awareness of his own splendid uniqueness in that he sticks out of nature with a towering majesty, and yet he goes back into the ground a few feet in order blindly and dumbly to rot and disappear forever. It is a terrifying dilemma to be in and to have to live with.[1]

Becker's dualistic thinking, and his view of death, are both open to criticism from philosophical and theological points of view.[2] But this should not detract from the analytic power of his notion of the existential paradox. Becker calls attention to a dialectic within human beings' self-awareness. He captures the tension arising from the experience of living on the boundary.

I want to stress the ways that people with chronic illnesses and disabilities live on this boundary. In what I would call "the existential paradox of chronic illness," people with chronic conditions are impelled at once to defy limitations in order to realize greater life possibilities, and to accept limitations in order to avoid enervating struggles with immutable constraints. This is the dialectical nature of chronic illness and disability. Their existential challenge is, to paraphrase Kierkegaard, the synthesis of possibility and necessity. Yet this is also the dialectic of hoping, which, as Marcel observed, always presupposes the temptation to despair.

In taking chronic illness and disability as a context for exploring the dynamics of hoping, I intend to cast some new light on both the experience of chronic conditions and the experience of hope. I will begin by elaborating my understanding of the existential paradox of chronic illness. I will then shift to an analysis of the dynamics of hoping as they appear from perspectives in social psychology and existential phenomenology. I will conclude by suggesting that these perspectives converge on several elements of hoping that bear directly on the experience of living with chronic conditions.

Before I begin, I want to say explicitly what is already implicit in this introduction. The dialectical nature of chronic illness and disability, especially the existential challenge of living on the boundary between finitude and transcendence, is a *human* problem, not a problem of the chronically ill or disabled person alone. If I have also set it as an intellectual "problem" in this essay, I do so not simply as an intellectual exercise, or even as an effort to "contribute" to our understandings of illness and medical care. I do not see myself primarily as a "contributor" here.

I am inviting people to join not only in my fascination with the dynamics of hoping, but in what I take to be a common human search for the grounds and possibility of hope.

The Existential Paradox of Chronic Illness

The aspect of chronic illness and disability that I am trying to evoke is expressed in the words of Alice Alcott (not her real name), whose experience with severe cardiovascular complications of diabetes forms part of Arthur Kleinman's study, *The Illness Narratives*.

> Time is running out for me, doctor. For others there is hope of cure. But for me this disease can never go away. The complications get more severe. The losses are greater. Soon, if not now, there will come a time when those losses are so great I will not want to bounce back. . . . If not now, then next week, next month, next year—things will be worse again. In the meantime, what is there for me: no left foot, a bad heart, poor circulation even to my good leg, failing vision. Parents I can't take care of, children for whom I'm unavailable. A husband as exhausted and despondent as I am. Myself, doctor, facing the long downhill road. Perhaps speaking to you will help me now, but can it change that road? No! I will do my best again to fight back. I will try to get on top of this thing. Yet in the long run, I will go down that road myself. Neither you nor anyone else can prevent it, or control it, or understand it for me. Can you give me the courage I need?[3]

Here is the tension, the inner dialectic of chronic illness and disability: *I will do my best again to fight back. I will try to get on top of this thing. Yet in the long run, I will go down that road myself.* Simultaneously, Alice Alcott experiences herself as imprisoned by her disease, and as battling against it. She is striving to stave off the destiny her condition has decreed, even as she recognizes its inevitability.

Kleinman's term for the process of kindling hope in individuals like Alice Alcott is "remoralization." It suggests the recovery of courage and hopefulness that have been lost through the *de*-moralizing confrontation with unavoidable limitation and loss. The tension between remoralization and demoralization is another way of expressing the intimate connection between hope and despair; it is the emotional counterpart to the more abstract, metaphysical concept of reconciling possibility and necessity. Complete demoralization would signal a capitulation to necessity that excluded any sense of possibility—there would be, in Alice Alcott's terms, no "trying to get on top of this thing." On the other hand, a remoralization that completely banished the enduring reality of limitation and loss would be an embrace of possibility that denied necessity—there would be no awareness of having "to go down that road myself."

Irving Zola has evoked some further dimensions of the existential paradox. Zola's studies of the social and psychological aspects of illness and health care merged with his autobiography when he spent a week living at Het Dorp, a community in The Netherlands designed to maximize possibilities for independent living for people with significant physical disability. Zola contracted polio and subsequently had a serious automobile accident, all between the ages of fifteen and twenty. These events left him with significant disabilities of his own. But it took his experience of living at Het Dorp as a participant-observer to make Zola aware that his adaptation to those disabilities had entailed a refusal to integrate them into his sense of himself:

> The very process of successful adaptation not only involves divesting ourselves of any identification with being handicapped, but also denying the uncomfortable features of that life. Not to, might have made our success impossible! But this process has a cost. One may accept and forget too much. Frankly, Het Dorp made me remember much more than I might have wished.[4]

What Alice Alcott experienced as an orientation toward her future, Zola here evokes as an orientation toward his past and present—as a question of personal identity. *One may accept and forget too much.* My interpretation of Zola's words is that in terms of identity the person with a chronic condition is pulled toward two extremes. In one direction, he or she may become wholly identified with the impaired self, feeling no access to any part of the self that is independent of impairment, in which case one has "accepted too much." In the opposite direction, the identification is *only* with the part of the self that is free of impairment, thereby "forgetting too much," to the exclusion not only of one's limitations but of one's grief and anger at those limitations, which are also part of one's identity.

A third dimension of the dialectic of chronic illness and disability lies in the sense of connection to the world. Persons with chronic conditions are often pulled in the contrary directions of self-protective withdrawal from, or eager participation in, the world of the "normals." Robert F. Murphy, who described his ten-year, progressive paralysis from a slowly growing spinal tumor in the book *The Body Silent*, characterized this tension as "the battle of life's wounded against isolation, dependency, denigration, and entropy, and all other things that pull them backward out of life into their inner selves and ultimate negation."[5] At one level the tension arises out of one's tendency either to accept or to resist messages of denigration and rejection from the social world. At another level it stems from the physical, institutional, and bureaucratic barriers by which society marginalizes people who have impairments of one sort or another, and from the sheer effort it can take—largely because of these barriers—just to get around.

But the tension between connection and separation is even more fundamental. Murphy, for example, makes use of the concept of "liminality" to describe the long-term physically impaired individual:

> They are human beings but their bodies are warped or malfunctioning, leaving their full humanity in doubt. They are not ill, for illness is transitional to either death or recovery. . . . The sick person lives in a state of social suspension until he or she gets better. The disabled spend a lifetime in a similar suspended state. They are neither fish nor fowl; they exist in partial isolation from society as un-defined, ambiguous people.[6]

Part of the experience of chronic illness and disability is the need to take a stance toward the world, rather than simply being able to take participation in the world for granted as a given of one's existence. Writing of those with a physical disability, Zola puts the matter sharply:

> Born for the most part into normal families, we are socialized into that world. The world of sickness is one we enter only later, poorly prepared and with all the prejudices of the normal. The very vocabulary we use to describe ourselves is bor-rowed from that society. We are de-formed, dis-eased, dis-abled, dis-ordered, ab-normal and, most telling of all, called an in-valid. And almost all share deep within ourselves the hope for a miracle to reverse the process, a new drug or op-eration which will return us to a life of validity.[7]

Return us to a life of validity. With this phrase Zola suggests that what is at stake in coming to terms with chronic illness and disability—in a world that construes these conditions as abnormal and those who have them as less than fully human—is not only the accomplishment of this or that particular goal, but the validity of one's very existence. Given this social construction, chronic illness and disability do not simply make specific aspects of daily living more difficult or complicated. They create a rift in the most basic sense we have of ourselves as persons in the world. They give rise to an awareness of separation or alienation. The tension within the experience of chronic conditions lies in the uncertainty whether this separation or alienation can be reduced. On one side are the stubborn day-in day-out realities of limitation and dependency. On the other side are all the energies and talents people draw upon to imagine and fulfill their potential. On the boundary, in the dialectic of possibility and necessity, is precisely where we would expect to encounter the dynamics of hoping.

Perspectives on Hope from Social Psychology and Existential Phenomenology

Physicians from Hippocrates to Osler have praised the positive effects of hope, without ever dwelling on the actual processes of hoping. More recent investigations have usually lumped hope together with all sorts of other positive mental states—e.g., optimism, faith, trust, a sense of agency or internal control—without differentiating among them or delineating the particular characteristics of hope. It is important to note that hope is itself a boundary concept. It belongs to no single intellectual discipline. Philosophers, theologians, psychologists, and sociologists have all claimed it within their province. In my discussion I will draw particularly on the work of three people: the social psychologist Shelley Taylor, and Gabriel Marcel and Paul W. Pruyser, who write from the perspectives of existential phenomenology. Though these are very different frameworks, taken together they capture elements of hoping that bear significantly on the dialectical nature of chronic illness and disability.

Shelley Taylor and the Theory of Cognitive Adaptation

Shelley Taylor begins with this observation:

One of the most impressive qualities of the human psyche is its ability to withstand severe personal tragedies successfully. Despite serious setbacks such as personal illness or the death of a family member, the majority of people facing such blows achieve a quality of life or level of happiness equivalent to or even exceeding their prior level of satisfaction.[8]

Taylor studied a number of women with breast cancer. In her interviews she encountered three recurring themes in the women's accounts of coping with the news of their disease: a search for meaning, an attempt to regain mastery over the events of their lives, and an effort to enhance their self-esteem. It was especially striking to Taylor that the means by which these women attempted to accomplish these goals involved some predictable modifications in their views of reality.

The cognitions upon which meaning, mastery, and self-enhancement depend are in large part founded on illusions. Causes for cancer are manufactured despite the fact that the true causes of cancer remain substantially unknown. Belief in control over one's cancer persists despite little evidence that such faith is well placed.

Self-enhancing social comparisons are drawn, and when no disadvantaged person exists against whom one can compare oneself, she is made up.[9]

The women in Taylor's research who appeared to be coping most constructively with their cancer expressed unjustified certainty as to the cause of their disease; they exaggerated their ability to control the progress of their disease and events in their lives generally; and they expressed self-appraisals that appeared to clash significantly with the "objective" severity of their physical, social, or economic circumstances. These women were sustained, Taylor argues, by unrealistically positive views of themselves, their personal control, and their ability to perceive order and meaning in events—in other words, by *illusions*.

Though these perceptions were unrealistic, they often contributed to bringing the distorted view of reality closer to the truth. The more positive views were energizing. They instilled persistence and a willingness to strive against obstacles. They gave confidence in social situations and thus helped bring about the very situations that were likely to enhance self-esteem. "The effective individual in the face of threat," Taylor concludes, "seems to be one who permits the development of illusions, nurtures those illusions, and is ultimately restored by those illusions."[10]

But there is a problem. As Taylor herself notes, theories of positive mental health have almost unanimously included accurate perception of reality as a cardinal element. After all, if we defend ourselves from life's negativities by wrapping ourselves in positive illusions, how can we ever learn from bad experiences? (Indeed, to return to the medical context, physicians often try to dispel their patients' illusions, in the belief that people are better off when they "face facts.") And there is a further problem. What happens when distorted perceptions of reality *are* disproved by experience? If positive illusions are helpful adaptive mechanisms in the face of threat, what happens to one's adaptation when the illusions that sustain it must yield to the way things "really are"?

These two questions—the role of illusions in positive mental health, and how one can simultaneously benefit from positive illusions and respond realistically and appropriately to negative information—have been at the center of Taylor's research for the past decade.[11] They are directly related to our question about chronic illness, disability, and hope. Consider the themes from the preceding section: envisioning the future; conceiving oneself as a social being; incorporating agency and autonomy as well as impairment in one's sense of self. These are closely related to Taylor's themes of meaning, mastery, and self-esteem. At issue in both contexts is the ability to derive energy and strength from the products of one's imagination without taking flight into frankly delusional thinking or ignoring the demands of everyday reality. In short, Taylor has expressed in social-psychological terms the existential challenge of hoping: the synthesis of possibility and necessity.

Using the concepts and language of social cognition theory, Taylor and her colleagues have defined the problem this way:

> If illusions are particularly functional when a person encounters negative feedback, we must consider, first, how the process of rejecting versus accommodating negative feedback occurs, and, second, how people negotiate the world successfully and learn from experience without the full benefit of negative feedback.[12]

To answer these questions, Taylor distinguishes illusion from repression and denial. In her usage, repression and denial refer to the *alteration* of reality, whereas illusions are primarily a *reinterpretation* of reality in accord with preferences or needs. People who rely on illusions (as opposed to denial) take maximum advantage of the ambiguous elements in most life situations and make interpretations of reality that give themselves "the benefit of the doubt."[13] People who rely on positive illusions also appear to have better social and interpersonal skills than people who depend on strong denial and repression. This seems to be related to the more global control of emotions that is associated with denial as compared to illusion. People who rely on denial or repression when dealing with negative situations typically display an absence of both positive and negative emotions. Illusions, on the other hand, tend selectively to mute negative affect.

Illusions are similarly selective in their openness to negative but potentially useful information. Whereas denial and repression typically increase in strength and rigidity as a threat increases, illusions are more flexible. Illusions permit a more subtle responsiveness to information, filtering and sorting feedback from the environment while permitting information necessary for learning to enter awareness. Unlike denial and repression, which block information and inhibit learning, illusions allow interpretations of reality that are more likely to remain within adaptive bounds.

According to Taylor, the flexibility of cognitive style that is associated with illusions is the key to their adaptive value. This flexibility manifests itself in several ways. Negative information may be filtered out to the extent that it is trivial, or short-term in its implications. More significant information, with greater potential impact on the person, is brought into awareness. Or, information that reflects badly on the self may be identified with a particular *part* of the self, but be prevented from influencing one's self-concept in a global fashion. This part of the self can then be interpreted as distant from one's "core" or "essential" nature, further minimizing the impact of the negative information on self-esteem.

Some events, of course—including severe chronic illness or disability—are simply too powerful and pervasive in their impact to be dealt with by these strategies. And yet Taylor wishes to argue that it is precisely these sorts of situations that lend themselves to the ameliorating effects of positive illusions. She suggests that in situations of extreme or pervasive threat, people who adapt constructively tend to be those who can reorient themselves to those spheres of activity or self-esteem that continue to be responsive to their efforts. For example, while one's view of the future, of one's self, or of the benevolence of the world may be strongly shaken by disease or disability, one may still retain the ability to define personal priorities or to improve personal relationships. The ability to make this type of shift, and to allow energizing, self-enhancing illusions to have their effect in whatever domains of life remain hospitable to them, is at the heart of the adaptive process.

Finally, Taylor makes an observation that is very much in keeping with the notion that hope involves existing on a boundary. Illusions, she points out, neither totally remove us from the world we live in, nor simply reinforce the constraints and limitations of that world. Even in the face of global threats, positive illusions can be at least partly self-fulfilling. They promote the energy for persistent striving. They distract us from obsessive brooding about slights or disappointments that don't really matter. They sustain the courage for social interactions that can lead to enhanced self-esteem, as well as to the achievements that result when people work together. In short, illusions can be instrumental in "creating the world that we believe already exists."[14]

Marcel and Pruyser on the Phenomenology and Metaphysics of Hoping

The approach to the dynamics of hoping represented by Marcel and Pruyser seems far removed from the work of Shelley Taylor. Where Taylor makes extensive use of her own and others' empirical research, Marcel and Pruyser proceed primarily by way of introspection, philosophical and theological reflection, and, especially in Pruyser's case, reference to psychoanalytic ego psychology and object relations theory. Marcel even insists that hope is a "mystery," not a "problem," and the attempt to pin it down with precise, rationalistic categories or empirical descriptions inevitably results in flattening out and distorting our understanding of it. Nonetheless, the juxtaposition of these perspectives will be fruitful for two reasons. First, the different methods and assumptions of existential phenomenology disclose subtle elements of hoping that we would otherwise miss. And, for all their differences, these approaches actually lead to some striking convergences, with interesting implications for understanding the experience of living with chronic illness and disability.

On one issue these approaches coincide exactly, and that is the dialectical tension within the dynamics of hoping. Whereas Taylor expressed this in terms of the need for positive illusions to permit realistic awareness of negative information from the environment, Marcel begins with the observation quoted in my epigraph, that hope exists only when there is the possibility of despair. Life is subject to being lived in hope just insofar as life is apt to be experienced as a "captivity." It is impossible to separate genuine "hope" from the framework of a "trial," that is, some experience of darkness, illness, separation, or slavery to which hoping is a response.[15]

From here, however, Marcel's approach diverges from that of most psychologists. He asks us to consider the difference in tone and meaning between the expression "I hope . . . " and the expression "I hope that. . . . " The latter phrase really expresses a concrete *wish*: I hope that I recover; I hope that I get the scholarship; I hope that I make it to high ground before the floodwaters overtake me. These "hopes" are more properly seen as ardent wishes. They are specific and concrete goals we are striving to achieve, and the strength of the "hope" is determined by the perceived value to us of the object of our desire. It is further characteristic of wishing (as opposed to hoping) that the self—with its needs, desires, or demands—is very prominent. This usage of "hope" is actually quite consistent with most of the social-psychological literature, which typically defines hope as the positive expectation of realizing desirable outcomes.[16]

Marcel, by contrast, stresses that hope transcends the particular objects or goals to which it may at first seem attached, and that in hoping the self is less at the center of attention. Hoping is a posture, not a motive for the achievement of a particular goal. It is a mode of experiencing oneself in relation to reality and time.

Hoping expresses an openness to novelty, possibility, and surprise—to "the mysterious reality which surrounds and at the same time confronts us."[17] In Pruyser's words, hoping means "surrender, not only to reality-up-till-now, but also to reality-from-now-on, including unknown novelties."[18] While the "realist" sees things only as they are, and rather narcissistically asserts that he or she *knows* that this is "the way it is," the hoper sees "experience-in-formation," modestly acknowledging that all has not been revealed to us.

Hoping is the enemy of fixity. It introduces a fluidity and even a playfulness into our constructions of the world. Hoping, Pruyser suggests,

> is not denial of reality, but a continued reevaluation of its content in contrast to other possible evaluations. From a structural point of view one might also say that at the moment hoping sets in, the hoper begins to perceive reality as of larger scope than one he has hitherto dealt with.[19]

To hope means to project oneself beyond one's present definition of reality, but with no guarantees against disappointment. Hoping thus takes on the risk inherent in finitude, including the finiteness of our formulations of reality itself. Despair, on the other hand, concretizes and eternalizes the present, and views time only as the ceaseless reiteration of one's captive state. Viewed in this light, despair appears to be a defense against the very risk of disappointment that hope takes on. To reject hope minimizes the risk of depending on a new and therefore unfamiliar vision of what is possible. It is the strategy that Paul Tillich described as avoiding being in order to avoid the threat of non-being.[20]

In the concrete context of chronic illness, the temptation to "avoid being" in order to avoid the risks and disappointments inherent in disability and limitation can be very strong. Retreat and withdrawal can seem to be the safest, most desirable response to the ceaseless challenges of living with physical impairment. Robert Murphy experienced this temptation as "a profound and deepening sense of tiredness—a total, draining weariness that I must resist every waking minute." Acknowledging that everyone experiences the desire to pull back from the hurly-burly of living from time to time, Murphy insists that "the deeply impaired harbor these urges chronically, sometimes because they are depressed but more often because they must each day face an inimical world, using the limited resources of a damaged body."[21]

Murphy goes on to reiterate the dialectical tension in the experience of chronic illness, the dialectic that I have attempted to delineate within the experience of hoping as well:

> Many give in to the impulse to withdraw, retreating into a little universe sustained by monthly social security checks, a life sustained by the four walls of an apartment and linked to outside society by a television set. . . . Many other disabled people go forth to battle the world every day, but even they must wage a constant rear-guard action against the backward pull. This is a powerful centripetal force, for it is commonly exacerbated by an altered sense of selfhood, one that has been savaged by the partial destruction of the body.[22]

Where the Perspectives Converge: Hoping and the Play of the Imagination

Though the two approaches to the dynamics of hoping that we have been examining are very different, both focus on hope as a *way of perceiving* that sustains creative striving in the face of adversity. For Taylor the main object of perception is the self: its worth, its ability to exercise control, its convictions of meaning and purpose. Using a host of cognitive mechanisms, the hopeful person continually readjusts his or her self-image. The goal is to make necessary accommodations to reality while maintaining a state of positive motivation. For Marcel and Pruyser, hoping involves perceptions of reality and time. Reality is seen as fluid and in-process; time is experienced as the realm of novelty and discovery. In their analysis the hopeful person, rather than being defined (or enslaved) by particular wishes, is continually open to the possibility that reality will disclose as yet unknown sources of meaning and value.

The emphasis on hoping as a mode of perception explains the significance for both approaches of the concept of *illusion*. Taylor and Pruyser, especially, lay great stress on illusion in their analyses of hope. A deeper understanding of this term will lead us to the heart of the dynamics of hoping.

The key element in Pruyser's view of illusion is the Latin *ludere*—to play—that is its etymological root. Inspired by the theories of Winnicott, Hartmann, and Erikson, Pruyser posits three realms of cognition, not two. Between primary process and secondary process, between hallucination and hard facts, between autistic and realistic thought, lies a third sphere—the *illusionistic sphere*. This is the realm of play, culture, and imagination. In this sphere there is constant interplay between internal images and external objects, between personal gropings toward meaning and the affirmations and corrections of culturally available formulations. The illusionistic world is the realm of symbols and of the products of human creativity, including art and religion.[23]

I would like to follow Pruyser's lead and suggest that hope is a product of the "play" of the imagination. In so doing I mean to exploit the gamut of associations that are attached to this word. Playing means to experiment in one's imagination with alternative pictures of reality. In play we fashion and refashion pictures and stories of the future. When we play we are not bound to the present circumstances of reality as it is. Instead, our play reflects the creativity of our imagination applied to reality as it might become. "Play" also means "give" or "flexibility," as in "there is play in the rope." Recall Taylor's idea that people continually rearrange their priorities, and consequently their definition of core features of the self, in the face of overwhelming negative feedback from the environment.

To hope is to adopt a playful attitude to reality, time, and the self. Yet there is an element of risk in playing, as there is in hoping. In both playing and hoping we project ourselves beyond what is familiar, toward what is new. As I have suggested, the avoidance of risk may account for the perverse attractiveness of despair, which by concretizing and eternalizing the present surrounds us with the comfort and safety of the known.

In summary, the dynamics of hoping involve three principal elements, all of which are embedded in the concept of play: imagination, movement, and risk. When we hope we detach ourselves from the story of our lives up to now. We imagine new stories and draw new pictures of our world, envisioning ourselves within those pictures. There is movement in this process of detachment from one story line, or picture, followed by attachment to another. The risk is that, having moved away from familiar stories and pictures, we must exist in a period of transition wherein we recognize the inapplicability of the old story, but have not yet become convinced of the coherence or even the direction of the new one. The hopeful person is on the boundary between old formulations of the self and new formulations not yet born.

What sustains us on this boundary? I would suggest that it is our experience of relationship, and our sense of connection to a sustaining spiritual environment and to a wider social world. It is the recognition that we do not create and re-create ourselves totally afresh, with only the resources that we invent. Personal identity is a synthesis of our own values and aspirations with the possibilities and constraints of our cultural and historical situation. The forms and images that animate the illusionistic sphere are not purely individual or intrapsychic products; nor are our assertions of hopefulness merely cast into a void.

In Marcel's terms,

> The essential problem to which we are seeking to find the solution would be whether solitude is the last word, whether man is really condemned to live and die alone, and whether it is only through the effect of vivid illusion that he manages to conceal from himself that such is indeed his fate. It is not possible to sit in judgment on the case of hope without at the same time trying the case of love.[24]

Hoping is a social and not merely a psychological phenomenon. *It is not possible to sit in judgment on the case of hope without at the same time trying the case of love.* Human beings are embedded in historical, cultural, and interpersonal structures that supply symbolic forms for the play of the imagination. These structures also provide validation for our expressions of hope.[25] At the social and cultural level, this is the function of religious narratives of hope and of the forms of communal participation through which these narratives are transmitted and reinforced. At the interpersonal level, part of the inspiriting power of hoping is the affirmation and confirmation that comes from having our hopefulness mirrored back to us in the empathic responses of others. The very act of inventing and telling new stories, in other words, implies that someone is there to hear them. An environment that cannot or will not hear our stories is an environment that is inimical to hoping.

Chronic Illness and the Dynamics of Hoping

Midway through *The Illness Narratives*, Arthur Kleinman pauses to imagine his readers' reactions to his stories of loss, limitation, and pain. He wants to balance the picture. He wants to remind his readers that the lives of many people with severe chronic illness and disability are models of "mastery and grace under fire," to demonstrate that it is possible to "maintain one's aspirations in the face of grave adversity."[26] In short, Kleinman wants to write about chronic illness, disability, and hope.

Interestingly, the story Kleinman tells to illustrate hoping in chronic illness (the story of Paddy Esposito)[27] is one that he himself acknowledges is so exceptional that he doubts most of his other patients, or students, could relate to it. Indeed, Kleinman offers remarkably little commentary on Paddy Esposito's story, and little analysis of hope. His economy is all the more striking in comparison with the extensive commentary he provides on other cases and his elaborate development of other concepts. What Kleinman does say is important—the need to understand hope in the context of an individual's concrete experience; the typical oscillation between hope and despair, rather than hope as a once-and-for-all achievement—but it is sparse. His message seems to be that in the presence of hope the best we can do is tell stories about it, let the particularities shine through, and refrain from analyzing it.

This may be the most appropriate response. After all, we have already been warned by Marcel that hope is a mystery, not a problem, and that we risk distorting it by making it the object of conceptual and empirical study. Nonetheless, I believe the preceding analysis does bring to light important dimensions of the experience that Kleinman wants to portray. I observed earlier, for example, that Kleinman frequently uses the term "remoralization" to refer to the process of maintaining one's aspirations in the face of adversity. I believe that the dynamics of hoping I have discussed lend greater psychological and spiritual content to Kleinman's terminology. They suggest some of the processes that may be at work as people move from the demoralizing encounter with limitation and loss to the recovery of hope and courage. Beyond this, I want to suggest how the dynamics of hoping relate to two other ideas that are fundamental to Kleinman's discussion of chronic illness and the care of the chronically ill: the idea of *the illness narrative*, and the idea of *empathic witnessing* as the crucial therapeutic response.

Before proceeding, however, I would recall my introductory comment that analyzing hope in the context of chronic illness and disability promises to throw new light not only on chronic conditions but also on hope. Certain features of the experience of chronic illness and disability pose critical questions for the preceding theoretical analysis. We need to consider these questions before we make use of the analysis in further elucidation of that experience.[28]

One question concerns the interpretation of hoping as primarily an orientation toward the future. For the person with a chronic illness or disability—particularly if the condition is progressive—it is precisely the future that is most uncertain and most threatening. This suggests two refinements in our initial formulation. The first is greater emphasis within the experience of hope on *continually shifting* time horizons, between the sort of openness to novelty and change that is evoked by Pruyser and Marcel, and a focus on the here and now that facilitates creative striving relatively independent of any sense of the future. The second is greater stress on the dialectical tension between hope and despair. As Kleinman suggests, this is more typical of people's experience than is any sort of once-and-for-all attainment of hope. This oscillation will in part reflect the changing coloration and immediacy of the sense of the future that a person has at any given time.

Another question concerns the contrast between hoping and wishing. Though specific wishes may be contrary to the experience of hoping as interpreted existentially and phenomenologically, aiming to achieve particular goals can make the otherwise overwhelming challenges of disabling conditions seem more manageable. The ability to formulate and pursue wishes is also part of the hopeful person's creative response to his or her situation. Once again we are led to refine our understanding of hope in the direction of even greater emphasis on its dialectical nature. Just as hopeful people are likely to shift their time horizons, so are they likely to oscillate between an attitude of general expectant openness to the future and a focus on specific goals or wishes, despite the fact that Marcel and Pruyser explicitly contrast the latter with hope.

With these refinements in mind, let us now examine Kleinman's notions of the illness narrative and empathic witnessing in light of the dynamics of hoping. In the space of one page, Kleinman describes people with chronic conditions as historians, revisionist historians, interpreters, diarists, cartographers, critics, and myth makers.[29] Patients, he argues, rely on plots, core metaphors, and other rhetorical devices to order their experiences of illness. They transform the natural events of a disease into the personally significant events of a biographical narrative. It is the narrative that bears the *meaning* of an illness, a meaning (or more likely, meanings) fashioned out of culturally available images and symbols for expressing infirmity and suffering, as well as out of the very personal language spoken between individuals in a family.

The person with a chronic illness, then, tells a story. We might say more accurately that the illness experience—as opposed to the brute facts of the disease process—*is* a story. This "narratization" of illness is, in one sense, simply a manifestation of the narrative dimension of all human experience. But there are particular implications here for our understanding of hope. I suggested above that hope involves telling ourselves a new story. Through the play of the imagination we detach ourselves from the story of our lives up to the present and fashion alternatives. The dynamics of hoping in the context of chronic illness and disability thus amount to what we might call the "renarratization" of illness.

We can understand this renarratization in two ways. First, it can involve the reformulation of our image of the self and its possibilities. At this level, the new story we imagine involves us as the principal actor, and its scope is primarily that of our personal biography. At a broader, social level, however, the reformulation can take the form of a critique of the very categories by which society defines deviance and disability. Irving Zola, Adrienne Asch, Harlan Hahn, and others have stressed the social construction of disability.[30] People with disabilities and dependencies face many barriers to social participation, barriers that are physical, bureaucratic, and institutional. But *where* are these barriers, and *who* is responsible for them? To ask these questions opens the way to reformulating our understanding of the barriers, to seeing them as the results of political and economic choice, rather than as inherent in the individual's physical characteristics. This is to tell a very different *social* and *political* story, and to suggest very different avenues for change.

The second important concept in Kleinman's understanding of chronic conditions is empathic witnessing, which he defines as "the existential commitment to be with the sick person and to facilitate his or her building of an illness narrative that will make sense of and give value to the experience."[31] In the terms of our discussion, Kleinman is referring to the social dimension of hoping. Empathic witnessing most readily calls to mind the dyadic relationship between an individual patient and a caregiver. Indeed, this seems to be primarily what Kleinman has in mind. When there is someone to hear the new story that we have to tell, we experience an inspiriting confirmation and affirmation of our expressions of hope. Moreover, the presence of others—which can be communicated nonverbally (through touch, for example) as well as through attention to our stories—helps mitigate our anxiety in that uncertain time before we gain confidence in the coherence and direction of our new narrative-in-formation.

This dimension of hoping suggests a number of fascinating interactions between the participants in the dyad, with their mutual needs for the social reinforcement of hope. One example, which needs further study, is the interaction between the illusions and narratives of others—in which we may play a significant role—and our own. Do the illusions of others complement or complicate ours? Is our own hopefulness augmented or diminished as a consequence of the role we play in the other person's efforts to maintain hope?[32]

A second example is the infectiousness of hopelessness. It is well known that depressed or hopeless people can instill hopelessness in those around them, including their caregivers. (Chronically ill or disabled people being cared for by action-oriented professionals who thrive on dramatic results may be at special risk for this reaction.) Hopeless or frustrated caregivers are likely to withdraw from the source of their trouble, and in so doing to withhold the very element in the caring relationship—themselves—that can mitigate the hopelessness of the person in their care. A self-perpetuating cycle of withdrawal and mutually compounding hopelessness and isolation is set in motion.

As with renarratization, empathic witnessing also has a broader societal dimension. Social, cultural, and political responses to limitation and dependency shape individual experience and influence the possibilities for personal transcendence. Hoping is not merely an intrapsychic activity. It is the *interplay* of personal imaginative processes with the possibilities of one's historical situation, as these are made available and communicated through potent cultural symbols and social practices. In Zola's words,

> We must deal as much with social arrangements as with self-conceptions. One in fact reinforces the other. Thus, the problem of those with a chronic disability should be stated not in terms of individual defects and incapacities affecting our physical functioning, but in terms of the limitations and obstacles placed in the way of our daily social functioning. What should be asked is not how much it will cost to make a society completely accessible to all with physical difficulty, but

rather why a society has been created and perpetuated which has excluded so many of its members.[33]

The dynamics of hoping, therefore, point to the need not only for empathic interpersonal communication in the clinical setting, but also for the reassessment of societal responsibilities. They pose the question of the extent to which society and culture are hospitable to individuals' and families' demands for full participation and, in Zola's words, "a life of validity."

The relationship between self-conception and social arrangements leaves us with a final sense of the existential paradox of chronic illness. On one side is the drive toward self-reliance and toward transcendence of limitation through the force of our own imagination and will. On the other side is our ineluctable dependency on the responsiveness of the wider social world, and the more general way that hoping opens us to possibilities and powers beyond ourselves which are not at our command. For while hope is an important ingredient in action, hoping is not entirely an active process. Even our illusions are not simply a matter of personal choice. In addition to seizing a new standpoint toward ourselves and toward our future, there is in hoping the experience of *being grasped*. The experience of hope includes an element of quiet receptivity and even of surprise—an element captured in the theological concept of grace.

We are wont to try to reduce the tension between self-reliance and receptivity by denying our dependencies. A culture that celebrates autonomy and individuality encourages us in this direction. After all, there is vulnerability in receptivity, for there are no guarantees. As a response to this vulnerability, the conviction of self-sufficiency is a comforting illusion.

I have argued that hoping is intimately bound up with illusion. All illusions are not equally adaptive, however, and for persons with chronic illnesses and disabilities (or without) the illusion of total self-sufficiency may be among the most destructive. It not only cuts us off from very practical gains to be made in solidarity with others, it radically distorts our view of the human situation. With our self-sufficiency magnified, our vulnerabilities and dependencies blur and recede into the background. We lose sight of our existence on the boundary.

Acknowledgments

I am grateful to the participants in the seminar for many helpful comments and suggestions on the first draft of my essay. In particular I would like to acknowledge the help I received from Kay Toombs, Ruthanne Curry, Ron Carson, Lonnie Kliever, Sue Estroff, and Irving Zola.

NOTES

1. Ernest Becker, *The Denial of Death* (New York: Free Press, 1973), p. 26.

2. See, for example, Lucy Bregman, "Three Psycho-mythologies of Death: Becker, Hillman, and Lifton," *Journal of the American Academy of Religion*, 1984, 52(3): 461–479.

3. Arthur Kleinman, *The Illness Narratives: Suffering, Healing, and the Human Condition* (New York: Basic Books, 1988), pp. 38–39.

4. Irving K. Zola, *Missing Pieces: A Chronicle of Living with a Disability* (Philadelphia: Temple University Press, 1982), p. 206.

5. Robert F. Murphy, *The Body Silent* (New York: Henry Holt, 1987), p. 230.

6. Ibid., p. 131.

7. Zola, *Missing Pieces*, p. 206.

8. Shelley E. Taylor, "Adjustment to Threatening Events: A Theory of Cognitive Adaptation," *American Psychologist*, 1983, 38(11): 1161.

9. Ibid., p. 1167.

10. Ibid., p. 1168.

11. Shelley E. Taylor and Jonathon D. Brown, "Illusion and Well-Being: A Social Psychological Perspective on Mental Health," *Psychological Bulletin*, 1988, 103(2): 193–210; Taylor, et al., "Maintaining Positive Illusions in the Face of Negative Information: Getting the Facts without Letting Them Get to You," *Journal of Social and Clinical Psychology*, 1989, 8(2): 114–129.

12. Taylor and Brown, "Illusion and Well-Being," p. 201.

13. Taylor et al., "Maintaining Positive Illusions in the Face of Negative Information," pp. 117–118.

14. Ibid., p. 126.

15. Gabriel Marcel, "Sketch of a Phenomenology and a Metaphysic of Hope," in *Homo Viator*, trans. by Emma Craufurd (New York: Harper and Row, 1962), p. 30.

16. See, for example, C. R. Snyder et al., "Hope and Health," in C. R. Snyder and R. F. Donelson, eds., *Handbook of Social and Clinical Psychology: The Health Perspective* (New York: Pergamon, 1991), pp. 285–305; and C. R. Snyder et al., "The Will and the Ways: Development and Validation of an Individual-Differences Measure of Hope," *Journal of Personality and Social Psychology*, 1991, 60(4): 570–585.

17. Marcel, "Sketch of a Phenomenology and a Metaphysic of Hope," p. 59.

18. Paul W. Pruyser, "Phenomenology and Dynamics of Hoping," *Journal for the Scientific Study of Religion*, 1963, 3(1): 94.

19. Ibid., p. 92.

20. Paul Tillich, *The Courage to Be* (New Haven: Yale University Press, 1952). See especially pp. 64–70.

21. Murphy, *The Body Silent*, p. 90.

22. Ibid.

23. Paul W. Pruyser, "An Essay on Creativity," *Bulletin of the Menninger Clinic*, 1979, 43: 294–353; and *The Play of the Imagination: Toward a Psychoanalysis of Culture* (New York: International Universities Press, 1983). For a critical discussion of Pruyser's work that stresses these themes, see David Barnard, "Paul W. Pruyser's Psychoanalytic Psychology of Religion," *Religious Studies Review*, 1990, 16(2): 125–129.

24. Marcel, "Sketch of a Phenomenology and a Metaphysic of Hope," p. 58.

25. For further discussion of these points, see Erik H. Erikson, "Human Strength and the Cycle of Generations," in *Insight and Responsibility: Lectures on the Ethical Implications of Psychoanalytic Insight* (New York: Norton, 1964), pp. 111–157.

26. Kleinman, *The Illness Narratives*, p. 137.

27. Ibid., pp. 140–145.

28. I am indebted to Kay Toombs for raising the issues discussed in the next two paragraphs.

29. Kleinman, *The Illness Narratives*, p. 48.

30. See, for example, Zola, *Missing Pieces*; Adrienne Asch and Michelle Fine, *Women with Disabilities: Essays in Psychology, Culture, and Politics* (Philadelphia: Temple University Press, 1988); and Harlan Hahn, "Public Policy and Disabled Infants: A Sociopolitical Perspective," *Issues in Law and Medicine*, 1987, 3(1): 3–27.

31. Kleinman, *The Illness Narratives*, p. 54.

32. I wish to thank Ruthanne Curry for suggesting these questions.

33. Zola, *Missing Pieces*, p. 244.

❖ 4 ❖

RAGE AND GRIEF
Another Look at Dax's Case

LONNIE D. KLIEVER

MY FIRST ENCOUNTER with the remarkable story of Donald (Dax) Cowart was a viewing of "Please Let Me Die" in 1976.[1] That thirty-minute videotape had been shot two years earlier during Dax's treatment in the burn unit of John Sealy Hospital in Galveston, Texas. My reaction to the videotape was the same as virtually everyone who has ever seen it. I was equally stunned by the treatment scenes and the interview sessions. The videotape vividly depicts the debridement process, an extremely painful procedure wherein burn patients have dead tissue scraped off their wounds while being bathed in a whirlpool solution of warm water and Clorox. Punctuated by Dax's intermittent screams of protest and pain, the camera pans from his emaciated body to close-up shots of his raw wounds, his maimed hands, his scarred face, his graft-covered eye socket. In sharp contrast to these horrific treatment scenes, Dax later lies quietly in his bed and responds in a measured voice to Dr. Robert White's gentle questions about his reasons for wanting to die. Dax explains at some length why he does not want to go on living as a blind and crippled person. The contrast between those two scenes—between Dax frantically and Dax quietly protesting his situation—haunted me for years to come.

What amazed me most was the control that Dax exhibited in his bedside interview with Dr. White. There was no ranting against his fate or railing against his caregivers. Dax argued his reasons for wanting to die with remarkable dispassion if not detachment. The impression on the viewer was overwhelming: How could anyone doubt the sanity of this young man or the reasonableness of his wish to die? And yet there was a nagging feeling in my mind from my first viewing of the videotape that Dax was covering his feelings in his conversation with Dr. White. The very lack of affect in his voice suggested controlled rage rather than either rational detachment or drugged indifference as some have suggested. Even so, that suspicion merely deepened rather than tempered my horrified reaction to the Cowart story. Who wouldn't feel rage if they had found themselves confined to a body so badly wounded and so harshly treated?

What did surprise me six years later, when I began my work on the making of the film "Dax's Case," was the enduring power of Dax's rage.[2] From our first conversations, it seemed obvious to me that his interest in making an updated version of the videotape was fueled primarily by rage—by rage against the medical and legal professions, if not against his family and friends as well, for turning a deaf ear to his earlier pleas to be allowed to die. The depth and duration of that rage became obvious in the background research and the actual shooting of the film. Every one of Dax's doctors refers to his frequent and explosive outbursts of anger. His mother hints at the years of intense conflict following Dax's discharge from the hospital when she alone bore the burden of his care and the brunt of his rage. And Dax himself betrays his abiding anger by portraying himself during treatment as a prisoner of insensitive caregivers, if not a victim of malevolent torturers.

The Sources of Rage

What were the sources of Dax Cowart's original and enduring rage? In the film, Charles Baxter, who was Dax's primary care physician during his eight-month treatment at Parkland Hospital, believed that his repeated and stormy demands to die were the typical reactions of a burn patient to his extraordinary burden of pain and feelings of helplessness. Robert White, who was the consulting psychiatrist during his five-month stay in John Sealy Hospital, went further in describing his terrible outbursts as "little boy" feelings of rage against those who hurt him in the process of trying to heal him. Dr. White also noted that these explosive responses were complicated by unresolved oedipal conflicts between Dax and his mother. These portrayals of Dax's rage as temper tantrums might seem cogent for the extended period of his hospitalization. We can certainly understand how a person might regress to childish and even infantile patterns of behavior under crushing burdens of unrelenting pain and unrelieved helplessness.

Dax's medical records at the three hospitals where he received treatment over a fourteen-month period are filled with references to such stormy episodes of "acting out." His medical charts further note that on occasion he had to be restrained or isolated until he calmed down and got control of himself. Dax describes his own reaction to the pain of the Hubbard tankings in much the same way: "All I could do when I was returned to my room was scream at the top of my lungs until I passed out." He adds with forlorn recall, "And this went on day after day, week after week, month after month." Such explosive reactions are fully consistent with the dynamics of pain which are described in a growing medical, phenomenological, and autobiographical literature on the experience of bodily pain, especially chronic pain.[3]

Such emotionally charged reactions to pain are rooted in two dynamics of the experience of pain. In the first dynamic, experiences of severe and unrelenting pain often reorder the patient's familiar relationships between "self" and "body." Experiences of great pain are shocking reminders that the self depends on the body, that selves are radically contingent. For persons who are chronically ill, severely handicapped, or grossly disfigured, the body moves from the background to the foreground of their experienced world. Their culturally instilled sense of the transcendence of self over body collapses into either radical identification or radical alienation. Pain and illness can undercut the human being's capacity "to move out beyond the boundaries of his or her own body into the external, sharable world."[4] The body can literally become one's "world," as pain occupies more and more of one's consciousness and crowds out awareness of anything else. Or pain can have the opposite effect of destroying the human being's familiarity and unity with his or her own body. The body can become the enemy. "In illness the body is interposed between us and reality; it impedes our choices and actions and is no longer fully responsive. The body stands opposite to the self. Instead of serving us, we must serve it."[5] In either case, the person in pain is drawn toward the frustrating and infuriating world of infantile urgency and impotence.

The second dynamic of pain reinforces these experiences of radical bodily identification and/or alienation. Patients often experience the loss of their "voice," either in the literal sense of being unable to speak or in the cognitive sense of being unable to communicate. Elaine Scarry explores both aspects of pain's assault on language in her remarkable book *The Body in Pain*. On the one hand, pain resists linguistic expression: "Physical pain—unlike any other state of consciousness—has no referential content. It is not *of* or *for* anything. It is precisely because it takes no object that it, more than any other phenomenon, resists objectification in language."[6] But pain can also empty linguistic behavior: "Physical pain does not simply resist language but actively destroys it, bringing about an immediate reversion to a state anterior to language, to the sounds and cries a human being makes before language is learned."[7]

These two dynamics of physical pain are closely related to one another. By taking away the human voice, pain robs a person of the means both of transcending the body and of indwelling the body. Again, Scarry throws light on these inter-connections between pain, voice, and body in her phenomenology of torture.

> It is the intense pain that destroys a person's self and world, a destruction expe-rienced spatially as either the contraction of the universe down to the immediate vicinity of the body or as the body swelling to fill the entire universe. Intense pain is also language-destroying; as the content of one's world disintegrates, so the content of one's language disintegrates; as the self disintegrates, so that which would express and project the self is robbed of its source and subject.[8]

Thus, a clearer understanding of the power of intense pain to "unmake"—radi-cally—the suffering person's world helps us understand why Dax might have re-gressed to childish and even infantile patterns of behavior.

But this explanation throws little or no light on the anger that Dax still ex-presses years later over his past and present circumstances. Pain was and is a factor, but we must look deeper than Dax's remembered and continuing pain to under-stand his enduring rage. Let me state my thesis bluntly and then argue it at some length. In a word, Dax's rage then and later was rooted in grief. His volatile anger was triggered by stronger urges than rebellion, was fueled by deeper wounds than pain, was sustained by heavier burdens than helplessness. Dax's acting out was no mere "little boy" petulance born of frustration over physical suffering and psy-chological dependence. This was "grown-up" rage born of paralyzing grief—grief over the loss of his world and of his place in that world. No amount of pain killer and no manipulation of the clinical environment could have assuaged Dax's grief and thereby dispelled his rage.

This connection between rage and grief was first suggested to me by Robert A. Burt's book *Taking Care of Strangers.*[9] Long before the fuller Cowart story was known, Burt contended that Dax's insistent demands to die were something other than rational responses to his physical pain and helplessness. Paying more atten-tion to the words than to the images in Dr. White's videotaped interview, Burt detected more uncertainty than certainty, more despair than acceptance in Dax's demands to die. Not that Burt doubted for a minute that Dax really wanted to die. But he did have serious reservations over whether Dax's desire to die was his freely chosen wish or rather was a choice he felt others wanted for him. Burt believed that it was inevitable that Dax was struggling with deep feelings of guilt and shame—guilt over causing his father's death and shame over his loathsome con-dition. Either perspective could lead him to deepest despair. Either his guilt or his shame would raise profound doubts about whether he *deserved* to live, much less whether others wanted him to live. If these feelings were present, as Burt believes they were, Dax's expressed wish to die would have a very different meaning from its first appearance as a rational, self-determining act. That voiced wish would be either a bitter plaint of despairing abandonment or a desperate cry for moral reassurance.

Burt's efforts to understand the deeper dynamics of the Cowart story are certainly instructive. His attention to the power of such primitive feelings as guilt and shame is a timely warning against simply taking Dax's demand to die at face value. But neither feelings of guilt nor feelings of shame really explain the rage that accompanied Dax's original demands to die and that sustained his continuing insistence that he should have been allowed to die. Guilt or shame are feelings that more readily evoke despair rather than provoke rage. Of course, with nothing more than the videotape to go on, Burt was unaware of the terrible outbursts and smoldering anger that were portrayed in the later film. Little wonder that he saw despair rather than rage at work in Dax's wish to die.

I was at a loss myself for years to fully understand the rage that is documented in the hospital records and in the living memory of those who cared for Dax during his treatment and rehabilitation. Physical suffering or psychological immaturity seemed too obvious and too simple a way of explaining his extraordinary anger. Only recently did I find the key that opens a way to a fuller understanding of Dax's remarkable ordeal. Of all places, I found that key in a cultural anthropologist's report on his field work among the headhunting Ilongots of northern Luzon in the Philippines. Renato Rosaldo's primary concern in his book *Culture and Truth* is to present a new theory of social analysis which is more sensitive to the ways in which class, race, gender, and sexual orientation affect cultural meanings.[10] But it was Rosaldo's discovery of the connection between grief and rage among these Filipino headhunters that compelled him to rethink and remake social analysis.

In an extraordinary essay entitled "Grief and the Headhunter's Rage," Rosaldo explains how he was eventually driven to accept the headhunter's simple explanation of why he cuts off human heads. When asked why he takes human heads, an older Ilongot's answer was brief: "He says that rage, born of grief, impels him to kill his fellow human beings. He claims that he needs a place 'to carry his anger.' The act of severing and tossing away the victim's head enables him, he says, to vent and, he hopes, to throw away the anger of his bereavement."[11] To the Ilongot, grief, rage, and headhunting go together in a self-evident manner.

By Rosaldo's own testimony, he could not for the longest time accept that simple explanation. Both by training and by temperament, he was not prepared to accept either the cultural force of emotions or the literal descriptions of informants. Following the anthropological method of "thick description," he preferred to explore the richness and texture, to uncover the *multivocity* and *polyformity* of cultural symbols. Thus Rosaldo, assisted by his wife who was also an anthropologist, looked for "deeper" explanations of headhunting than the shallow one-line accounts offered by their Ilongot informants. He applied the "exchange theory" that dominates so many classical ethnographies, arguing that the victim of a beheading was exchanged for the death of one's own kin, thereby balancing the books. But Rosaldo's Ilongot informants refused to confirm this "deeper" reading of their reasons for taking human heads. They stubbornly stuck to their explanation that anger in bereavement was the only source of their desire to cut off human heads.

Just as stubbornly, Rosaldo stuck to his own exchange theory, even though his search for more verbal elaboration and analytical sophistication over the next two years merely reiterated the Ilongot's simpler reading. Rosaldo simply could not *imagine* the rage that can come with devastating loss. It took him fourteen years and a devastating personal loss to grasp what the Ilongots had told him about grief and rage. His preparation for understanding serious loss began with the death of his brother. Witnessing the ordeal of his mother and father, he gained some insight into the trauma of a parent's losing a child. But his bereavement was so much less than that of his parents that he still could not imagine the overwhelming force of rage possible in such grief. Only when he lost his wife to a terrible accident did he finally understand the sheer rage that grows out of grief.

In 1981, Rosaldo and his wife, Michelle, returned to the Philippines to begin field research among the Ifugaos culture. While walking along a trail with two Ifugaos companions, she lost her footing and fell to her death some sixty-five feet down a sheer precipice. Upon finding her body, Rosaldo became enraged. "How could she abandon me? How could she be so stupid?" Again and again in the months and years ahead, this tearless, numbing anger swept over him in a variety of forms, lasting hours and even days at a time. He experienced the deep cutting pain of sorrow beyond endurance, the cadaverous cold of the finality of death, the trembling emptiness of loneliness. For the first time he understood rage born of grief—a rage that can erupt like a sudden explosion or smolder like a hidden fire. And, for the first time he understood the headhunter's desperate need to find some place to "carry his anger," some way to "throw away his rage."

Rosaldo's inability to connect rage and grief among the Ilongots is typical for our North American culture. Middle-class Anglo-Americans especially tend to ignore the rage that devastating losses can bring.[12] Even though the work of grief therapists is widely talked about in our culture, the comforts of traditional religion and the conceits of enlightenment rationality alike still conspire to deny the explosive and enduring anger born of grief. The consolations of faith are expected to erase the grief in times of loss. The controls of reason are expected to defuse the rage in times of stress. Little wonder that neither Dax nor his caregivers were prepared to understand either the source or the force of his rage. For his caregivers, Dax's tremendous outbursts were infantile reactions to his pain and helplessness. Dax seems even less aware of the quality and intensity of his anger. He saw and sees his original demands to die as rational choices based on prudential considerations. But there is another way of reading the Cowart story that ties together Dax's original demands to die and his continuing resentment of those who refused those demands. Dax simply had no place to "carry his anger," no way to "throw away his rage."

The Solaces of Grief

Rosaldo's work with the Ilongots is instructive not only on the sources of rage but also on the solaces of grief. More to the point, Rosaldo's analysis suggests what can happen to the individual or group who finds no culturally sanctioned ways of dealing with grief. In 1972 the Ilongots faced an acute problem when headhunting was outlawed by the Marcos regime. The cessation of headhunting called for painful adjustments to other modes of coping with the rage they found in bereavement. Some Ilongots allowed their rage to dissipate, as best it could, in the course of everyday life. Many others began to convert to evangelical Christianity as a means of coping with their grief. On the one hand, accepting the new religion forced them to abandon their old cultural ways, including headhunting. On the other hand, it promised to make coping with bereavement less agonizing because they could believe their deceased had departed for a better world. But even those who converted to Christianity were filled with an enduring sadness because the old ways were no more. Indeed, the very stability of the society was shaken by the loss of their old way of dealing with rage and bereavement.

The intensity of Dax's rage can be grasped only when we understand the magnitude of his grief. Here we must understand that bereavement extends to any loss—the loss of love as well as life, the loss of work as well as health.[13] As Burt pointed out, Dax must have been grieved by the death of his father, who perished in the same conflagration that he survived. Dax's grief over his father's death might also be intensified by one fact of the accident: Donald Cowart turned the ignition switch that led to the explosion. No matter how irrational it might have been for him to feel guilty for that action, no matter how properly he had behaved toward his father throughout their relationship, no child can avoid feelings of recrimination in the wake of a parent's death.

Dax must also have been grieved by the reactions of others to his own woeful condition. He ruefully admits that being blind spared him the cruel stares of curiosity and horror from others. But Dax had to sense the discomfort and even disgust that others felt in his presence. He had to believe that others found him repelling and contemptible and that must have broken his heart. Finally, Dax must have grieved over the loss of his own life world—indeed, over the loss of his own identity. Quite apart from the crushing pain, Dax's sudden and total dependence on others radically undercut all sense of an identity separate from other people and from the external world. The fact of his blindness suddenly deprived him of a clear sense of the physical and social environment. His utter helplessness, which required others to move, feed, and toilet him like an infant, must have undermined his sense of power and worth. Dax could not help being overwhelmed by grief over these massive losses of self-care and self-worth. Art Rousseau explained Dax's wish to die in the film "Dax's Case": "He knew where he was coming from. He knew that he wasn't going to be Don Cowart any more!" In short, Dax was stricken with a triple burden of grief—the loss of his father, the loss of his companions, and the loss of himself.

That neither Dax fully acknowledged nor his caregivers fully understood his rage is evidence of how well our culture camouflages intense feelings growing out of death and disability. His episodes of rage were either trivialized as temper tantrums or dismissed as pain reactions. But explosive and simmering rage was surely there, precisely because Dax had no mythic or ritual way of freeing himself from his bereavement over his profound losses. Dax never addressed his situation, either in prospect or retrospect, from a traditional religious point of view. In defending his right to die, he appealed to specific legal canons of informed consent, to contemporary movements for civil rights, and to broad philosophical traditions of personal autonomy in explaining his behavior and defending his desires. But he nowhere invoked the Protestant heritage of his culture or the Church of Christ teachings of his childhood to interpret his experience, to ameliorate his suffering, or to support his views. Indeed, Dax's apparent rejection of his religious heritage goes deeper than either personal modesty about religious commitments or disaffection from religious institutions. His whole demeanor reflects a deep alienation from the central symbol and core of the Christian religion. Dax's approach to his own tragedy represents a categorical refusal of *redemptive* suffering.[14]

We search in vain for any echo of redemptive suffering in Dax's approach to his own pain and grief. He nowhere sees his accident as an occasion for deepening his spiritual relationship to God. He nowhere confronts his pain as the supreme test of his faith in the face of adversity. He nowhere resolves to conquer his handicaps in order to help others facing similar circumstances. He nowhere even defends his suicide attempts as an effort to relieve others from the burden of his care. Others in the film "Dax's Case" voice these possibilities for him. Dax's mother, Ada, prays that he will live long enough to come back to God. His physician, Duane Larson, dares him to get well and give life a try, and only then take his own life if things don't work out. Rex Houston, Dax's lawyer, encourages him to use the money he has been awarded to make something of his life. But Dax reaches for none of these ways of redeeming his own suffering from utter waste and despair.

With no culturally defined or personally validated way of "throwing away" his rage, Dax directed that rage at other targets. He focused his rage on those who provided him medical care—on doctors who treated him, on orderlies who forced him to walk, on nurses who changed his dressings. He vented his anger on his mother, who remained at his bedside for months during his treatment and cared for him during his years of rehabilitation. He directed his anger against impersonal institutions—toward lawyers who would not touch a case like his, toward hospitals that held patients hostage to expensive treatment procedures, toward society in general and civil rights movements in particular which celebrated individual rights for racial minorities but denied them to patients. Most of all, he turned his rage on his diminished self and especially on his contemptible body. Something of the intensity of that inward-directed anger can be gauged by the long years of chronic depression and the attempted suicides that dogged Dax after his discharge from the hospital.

Herein lay the pathos of the Cowart story, for Dax was neither allowed to die nor equipped to live by his caregivers.[15] He went years without reaching a positive alternative to the scheme of Christian redemptive suffering that he rejects. Those who have followed the Cowart story closely since the release of the film "Dax's Case" in 1985 are aware that rage—controlled but palpable—remained a driving force in Dax's life long after his terrible accident and harrowing rehabilitation. Indeed, hearing him speak to professional groups or reading his newspaper interviews left an indelible impression that Dax would never rest his "case" against those who saved his life and served his needs. For years he seemed to define his existence more by negation than by affirmation, more by death than by life. His memories were dominated by the unspeakable agonies that he suffered at the hands of uncaring tormentors. His expectations were darkened by the frustrations and limitations of his handicapped existence. Caught between bemoaning his survival and begrudging his existence, Dax seemed torn between life and death.

But Dax *has* continued on with his life. Indeed, he has achieved a quality of life far beyond what he or anyone else imagined possible, even during the years that "Dax's Case" was being filmed. Not that life has been easy for Dax and those around him. The business that he established and the marriage he entered during those years of the filming have long since failed. Although Dax subsequently returned to law school at Texas Tech University, where he completed his degree and passed the bar in the summer of 1986, the law practice that he established in his small East Texas home town has not thrived. Far from calling it quits, however, Dax continues to represent his views on patient rights at educational symposiums and public forums. He is married again, to a woman who seems to have brought a new measure of contentment into his life. Hearing him speak and talking with him as I have recently, I find that Dax displays a sense of humor and joy in living that simply were not there previously. When I pressed him about this change, Dax explained that he was trying to make the most of his life. He even offered what has become a secular credo of sorts, borrowed from self-help guru Anthony Robbins: "With every adversity comes the seed of an equal or greater opportunity."[16]

Given these tumultuous ups and downs, Dax's "case" vividly addresses many of the special problems faced by persons with disabling and disfiguring illnesses. Beyond the usual medical and legal aspects of acute medical crisis and care are the special problems of *chronic* illness and impairment: What are the sources of suffering for the chronically ill or permanently disabled patient? Does such illness engender its own distinctive kind of suffering? Do prevailing forms of medical care and social practice exacerbate these kinds of suffering? What makes the lived experience of chronic disease or permanent disability distinctively different from acute illness? What are the essential ingredients of a life worth living in spite of chronic illness and impairment? If health is not possible (in the sense of a life free from limitation, pain, and debility), what makes life meaningful? What medical care and legal options should be open to the chronically ill and impaired who cannot find any reason for going on with their lives?

The preoccupation of medical ethicists with treatment decisions arising out of situations of acute illness and imminent death has succeeded in pushing these questions—many of which are questions of *religious* meaning—to the side. We have spent our time and energy dealing with questions of medical frontiers, professional constraints, legal entitlements, and ethical guidelines in situations of emergency. We have left aside "the weightier matters of the law"—the medical, legal, moral, and religious guidelines for humane treatment and good care in situations of lasting physical and spiritual extremity. Is it any wonder that Derek Humphrey's *Final Exit* and Jack Kevorkian's "suicide machine" appeal to those who feel trapped in the "never land" of chronic illness and massive impairments? It is time we realized that questions of meaning—including how to deal with grief, how to dispose of rage—are just as important in systems of good care as are the usual medical, legal, and even moral issues.

The Relief of Suffering

Approaching "Dax's Case" as a "chronic illness" story rather than a "right to die" film will not be easy. The film itself is structured as a conflict between a patient who wanted to die and his family and physicians who would not let him or help him die. As one of the filmmakers, I can vouch for the fact that we tried to avoid tilting the "case" to one side or the other. But the sheer power of the visual images of Dax Cowart—before his accident, during his treatment, and after his rehabilitation—carries more weight than the viewer can dispassionately handle. The very *sight* of Dax Cowart stops argument dead in its tracks over whether he should or should not have been allowed to die. The viewer's mixed feelings of pity and revulsion at the sight of Dax's massive suffering and disfigurement are too overwhelming to hear any other voice in the film than his insistent demands that he wanted to die. The voices of family, friends, nurses, and especially doctors are drowned out by the cries in the treatment room, thereby silencing those very persons whose intimate ties to the patient would raise more sharply the question of whether he ought to kill himself and even whether he really wanted to die. To put it bluntly, "Dax's Case" *as viewed* has a protagonist but no serious antagonist. This one-sidedness is even more overwhelming in the videotape "Please Let Me Die," where Dax is the only voice and where his ravaged body in treatment fills the screen from start to finish.

But for all of the dramatic and moral one-sidedness of the film as seen, "Dax's Case" can be viewed as a chronicle of tragic illness—tragic because neither Dax nor his caregivers fully recognized or acknowledged the deeper dynamics of his suffering. Curiously enough, this re-visioning of "Dax's Case" is prompted if not demanded by Dax's own continuing presence. The contemporary Dax Cowart, particularly the Dax Cowart who has appeared at many professional and academic presentations of the film, has almost unwittingly become his own antagonist. Viewers of the film where Dax is present are often torn between sharply conflicting emotions—outrage that this suffering man was not allowed to die and gratitude that this appealing person is still alive.

This typical reaction is documented in one of the earliest of Dax's many personal appearances.[17] John Lee Smith, a friend of mine and Dean of Students at the Cornell Law School who had used "Please Let Me Die" in the school's Program on Law and Ethics, learned of my work on a film sequel to this videotape. This discovery subsequently led to a fresh presentation of the Cowart Case at the 1983 Law School student retreat. On the first night, the script of the videotape (which was published in Burt's *Taking Care of Strangers*) was discussed by the students, who seriously questioned Cowart's sincerity and competence. A showing of the videotape the next morning evoked a widespread shift of opinion in support of, if not agreement with, Cowart's demand to die. But that evening Cowart appeared and interacted warmly and naturally with the group, raising new questions about what should or should not have been done with his demands to die. This was but the first of many occasions where the juxtaposition of Dax Cowart's living charm and disfigured body has exposed the deeper complexities and ramifications of the Cowart story.

Re-visioning "Dax's Case" in the way that I have suggested illumines a whole range of issues related to chronic illness and disability. I will concentrate here on the relief of suffering. For one thing, the Cowart story drives home the fact that such suffering is a *compound of pain and grief.* Everyone connected with Dax's care was mindful of his pain and its effect on his wish to die. Drs. Charles Baxter and Duane Larson acknowledge that burn patients undergo pain so excruciating that death looks like a welcome relief. Dr. Robert White sought to improve Dax's situation by treating his pain more aggressively, although these higher levels of pain medication did not completely dispel the agony. Looking back, Dax's mother believes that higher levels of pain medication would have made a difference in his will to live. Above all, Dax on occasion insists that pain was the driving force behind his wish to die. I certainly have no right or wish to minimize the terrible physical agony that Dax endured. But I am convinced, both on the basis of the film and by my wider familiarity with the Cowart story, that Dax's suffering was broader and deeper than physical pain alone. Dax's "suffering unto death" was compounded of pain and grief.

For purposes of emphasis, I have separated pain and grief in the foregoing re-visioning of "Dax's Case." I have thereby at least temporarily perpetuated what David B. Morris calls the "myth of two pains"—that physical and mental pain are divided into two types "as different as land and sea. You feel physical pain if your arm breaks. You feel mental pain if your heart breaks. Between these two events we seem to imagine a gulf so wide and deep that it might as well be filled by a sea that is impossible to navigate."[18] Like all cultural myths, this separation contains some serviceable truth. No one would wish to return to the more primitive theories of pain as demon possession or as vital humors. Yet in the long run, this nineteenth-century separation of pain into two radically different sources and valences has emptied physical pain of any meaning (It's only a neuroelectric impulse!) and deprived mental pain of any standing (It's all in your head!).

But an impressive variety of interdisciplinary pain studies and therapies are challenging this widespread myth. We are relearning scientifically and philosophically what all of us *know* for sure in the lived world of our own embodied existence. Put in simplest terms, when my heart aches my body hurts and when my body hurts my heart aches. Pain and grief are the Siamese twins of all human suffering. Pain and grief proceed together intertwined in such a way that it is impossible to *experience* them apart, however we may try to distinguish them in theory and in practice. Of course, short-term pain and grief create the illusion that they occur in logic-tight compartments, because we can bring them under control before they synergize. This separation is reinforced by the partial conquest of pain through a growing arsenal of medical analgesics. But the inseparability of pain and grief clearly emerges in cases of chronic illness and distress where there are no magic bullets to dispel suffering. Suffering is that mysterious process that binds body to mind and self to world. Suffering emerges at the intersection of bodies, minds, and cultures.[19]

Rightly viewed, "Dax's Case" confirms the medical and human tragedy of splitting human suffering into uncommunicating categories called physical and mental, or outer and inner. Dax's "case" might have had a very different outcome had those who cared for him been more sensitive to the full range and depth of his suffering. No one, perhaps with the exception of nurse Leslie Kerr and friend Art Rousseau, really saw through Dax's rage to the amalgam of pain and grief that tortured his body and anguished his heart. Either the grief was trivialized (Dr. Baxter's response to Dax's demands to die: "Ah Donnie, you don't want to do that") or the pain was magnified (Ada Cowart's explanation that Dax's demands to die were only "the pain talking"). But no regimen of care bent on actually relieving Dax's suffering and restoring his health could have succeeded without attending to both these dimensions of his profound illness and massive impairments. When the technical challenges of repairing the body are separated from the existential challenges of restoring the soul, the healing that does go on is incomplete and unsatisfactory. Had Dax been enabled to become a more courageous and cooperative patient, both his physical and his psychological outcome could have been substantially improved.

Moreover, "Dax's Case" reveals that suffering born of chronic illness and disability is an *assault on meaning and purpose*. Across all times and places, human suffering has been understood as an event that demands interpretation. Indeed, every religion if not every culture is a *theodicy*—a way of explaining and ameliorating human suffering. In the past, both pain and grief fell under the "nomizing" or ordering activity of culture:

> The individual is seen as being born, living and suffering, and eventually dying, as his ancestors have done before him and his children will do after him. As he accepts and inwardly appropriates this view of the matter he transcends his own individuality as well as the uniqueness, including the unique pain and the unique terrors of his individual experiences. He sees himself "correctly," that is, within the co-ordinates of reality as defined by his society. He is made capable of suffering "correctly" and, if all goes well, he may eventually have a "correct" death (or a "good death," as it used to be called). In other words, he may "lose himself" in the meaning-giving nomos of his society. In consequence, the pain becomes more tolerable, the terror less overwhelming, as the sheltering canopy of the nomos extends to cover even those experiences that may reduce the individual to howling animality.[20]

As such, human suffering was always physical and mental, always literal and symbolic, always personal and cultural.

But, as noted above, the nineteenth-century model of suffering has sundered pain and grief, thereby depriving pain of palpable meaning and grief of tangible reality. In modern medicine, the meaning of pain disappeared in biochemical processes and the reality of grief evaporated in psychological inwardness. To be sure, pain has been given a *scientific* explanation (which provides a meaning of sorts) and grief had been given a *scientific* status (which conveys a reality of sorts). But pain and grief without some *human* meaning and purpose casts us into a meaningless world. Suffering provokes a state of crisis. That crisis state involves more than physical discomfort. Suffering opens up a huge fissure in our world. Suddenly we do not possess the understanding we need. We need answers to incessant questions: Why is this happening to me? Why won't it stop? How will I ever earn a living if I'm disabled? Will my sex drive ever return? Am I doomed to spend the rest of my life in pain? We want to know what all this torment in our bones, all this chaos in our cosmos adds up to. What does it mean? Yet for all their urgent questions and devastating effects, conjoined pain and grief remain largely unrecognized by physicians and patients alike as constitutive aspects of all serious illness and impairment. Caregivers have yet to pay sufficient attention to the fact that chronic illness and impairment undermine life's fundamental meaning, values, and relationships.

That Dax was daunted by questions of the meaning and purpose of his suffering is evident in the film "Dax's Case." He deeply feared that his "incurable wounds" would cut him off permanently from the world of love and work. He despaired over "whether he would ever have a meaningful relationship with the opposite sex" or whether he could ever do more "than sell pencils on the street corner." His dreams no less than his body were shattered by that explosion that nearly took his life. Little wonder that his monumental grief and his massive pain sapped him of good reasons to go on living. While his caregivers were certainly not unaware of the depths of his despair, they were preoccupied with caring for his body to the neglect of curing his soul. To be sure, Dr. White sought to address these weightier problems during Dax's voluntary rehospitalization for acute insomnia and reactive depression in 1980. Indeed, Dax's "History and Physical Examination" taken at the time of his admission proposes to assist the patient "to resolve grief process and establish realistic life goals." That this goal of treatment was hardly realized at the time is a reminder that creating a new identity out of the ash heap of ruined aspirations and reduced abilities is an arduous and agonizing process. More important, the patient ultimately must take charge of his or her suffering and assume personal responsibility for its meaning.

Finally, "Dax's Case" reveals that suffering born of chronic illness and disability is an *obstacle to communication and communion*. Intense pain and grief can literally deprive the patient of voice. Such radical breakdowns in communication are due in part to the indescribability and unsharability of pain. They are also attributable to the paralyzing and alienating power of grief. But howling animality and sobbing abandonment are not the only ways those who are suffering lose their voices. The very breakdown of normal patterns of behavior, of assumed canons of meaning, of familiar relations of intimacy threatens to empty the patient's language of its taken-for-granted sense and reference. Serious illness and substantial disability can shock patients out of their commonsensical world. The patient must learn a new language that reorders as well as reflects his or her shattered world. That "re-making" requires far more than an internal dialogue. It involves reconnecting with the wider worlds of home and work, of family and society. Every meaningful relationship is changed as a consequence of the chronically ill or disabled patient's own altered existence.

Sad to say, the medical establishment often furthers the patient's loss of voice. Medicine is a foreign country filled with unfamiliar languages and customs, with complicated rights and duties. The patients' unfamiliarity with this alien world can intimidate them, leaving them virtually speechless. This breakdown of communication and communion between patient and healer is compounded by professional authoritarianism and paternalism. "Good" patients do what they are told to do by their doctors. "Good" doctors know what is best for their patients. This asymmetry of knowledge in the healing relationship results in a "power gap" between physicians and patients. Given these circumstances, the conspiracy of silence between physicians and patients which typifies most medical care is hardly surprising.[21]

But just as suffering has the power to destroy language, so language has the power to dissolve suffering. Freud's notion of a "talking cure" is not limited to psychological illness. Finding a language that leads the chronically ill and impaired out of their incomprehensible and inexpressible suffering plays a crucial role in overcoming that suffering. At its simplest level, this recovery of language involves objectifying the suffering as an identifiable pathology. At its most profound level, this restoration of voice involves transforming the suffering into purposeful activity. Neither of those tasks can be accomplished apart from a dialogical partnership between physician and patient. According to Jay Katz, that kind of dialogical interaction would restore the medical profession's exalted mission to heal humankind:

> The root meaning of doctor is "teacher" (from the Latin *docere*, to teach or to instruct), and the root meaning of physician is "a natural philosopher" (from the Greek *physicos*, an inquirer into nature). The two meanings must be joined so that physician-doctors can fulfill their dual functions as inquirers into the ills of mankind and patients, and as Socratic teachers who seek to arrive at a truth in concert with patients.[22]

On the face of things, the Cowart story is a classic case of autonomy versus paternalism. Certainly that clash is the perceived message of the film "Dax's Case" and represents Dax's own construal of his experience as a patient. But a more sensitive viewing of the film discloses that Dax was not totally without voice, particularly during the latter half of his treatment at the Institute for Research and Rehabilitation in Houston and at the John Sealy Hospital in Galveston.[23] To be sure, Dax only grudgingly admits that his refusal of the Hubbard tankings was finally honored in Houston and that no surgical procedures were performed in Galveston without his consent. Moreover, little is made in the film of the fact that Dr. White worked with Dax quite closely over a four-month period prior to his final discharge from John Sealy Hospital in August 1974. But, for the most part, no one wanted to talk openly and honestly with Dax about what he was undergoing. Whatever communication there was between Dax and his caregivers fell short of the full and frank medical and moral dialogue that might have changed the course of his treatment and the quality of his rehabilitation.

Summary

The kind of re-viewing of "Dax's Case" that I have suggested places this film among the growing number of "illness narratives" that have begun to reshape the field of medical ethics and the practice of medicine.[24] At the heart of this new attention to the patient's story is the recognition that the particular narratives of individual patients profoundly affect not only how they experience their illness but the course of that illness as well. The film "Dax's Case" illustrates what goes wrong when that narrative focus is ignored by either the physician, the patient, or, as in the Cowart story, by both. When illness and treatment are divorced from the patient's life story, the medical and moral issues are unavoidably reduced to technological-ethical decisions of the moment. Such quandaries are unavoidable in emergency rooms and intensive-care units. These situations require generalizable actions based on universalistic principles. But surely *patient* care (in both senses of that word) permits and requires a more individualistic treatment of illness that is informed by who the patient is and what suffering means to that particular person.

Seen as a narrative of illness, "Dax's Case" raises problems of a very different kind than if it is viewed as a "right to die" film. The relief of human suffering— suffering as a compound of pain and grief, suffering as an assault on meaning and purpose, suffering as an obstacle to communication and communion—lies at the center of those problems. It takes only half a turn to see Dax's demands to die as a struggle with life rather than as a surrender to death. Approached from this direction, the Cowart story becomes a paradigm case of the challenges and complexities, the shortcomings and failures of medical care for the chronically ill and disabled. We have as much to learn from Dax's case about the will to live as about the right to die.

NOTES

1. For a narrative summary of the Cowart story, see Keith Burton, "A Memoir: Dax's Case as It Happened," in *Dax's Case: Essays in Medical Ethics and Human Meaning*, ed. Lonnie D. Kliever (Dallas: Southern Methodist University Press, 1989), pp. 1–12.

2. The film "Dax's Case" is distributed by Filmaker's Library, 124 East 40th Street, New York, NY 10016.

3. For an annotated bibliography of these various approaches to pain, see David B. Morris, "The Languages of Pain," in *Exploring the Concept of Mind*, ed. Richard M. Caplan (Iowa City: University of Iowa Press, 1986), pp. 97–99.

4. Elaine Scarry, *The Body in Pain, The Making and Unmaking of the World* (New York: Oxford University Press, 1985), p. 13.

5. Edmund D. Pellegrino and David C. Thomasma, *A Philosophical Basis of Medical Practice: Toward a Philosophy and Ethic of the Healing Professions* (New York: Oxford University Press, 1981), p. 208.

6. Scarry, *The Body In Pain*, p. 5.

7. Ibid., p. 4.

8. Ibid., p. 35.

9. Robert A. Burt, *Taking Care of Strangers: The Rule of Law in Doctor Patient Relations* (New York: The Free Press, 1979).

10. Renato Rosaldo, *Culture and Truth: The Remaking of Social Analysis* (Boston: Beacon Press, 1989).

11. Ibid., p. 1.

12. Most recent anthropological studies of grief and mourning within traditional cultures acknowledge that anger and aggression are universal components of bereavement and show how these dangerous and disruptive responses to death and loss are controlled by ritual experts. But such ritualized opportunities for the controlled expression of anger and hostility have all but disappeared in modern cultures. See Colin Murray Parkes, *Bereavement: Studies of Grief in Adult Life*, Second American Edition (Madison, Conn.: International Universities Press, Inc., 1987), pp. 97–123; Paul C. Rosenblatt, R. Patricia Walsh, and Douglas A. Jackson, *Grief and Mourning in Cross-cultural Perspective* (New Haven, CT: Human Relations Area Files Press, 1976), pp. 13–17, 105–124; John S. Stevenson, *Death, Grief, and Mourning: Individual and Social Realities* (New York: The Free Press, 1985), pp. 121–168.

13. Not surprisingly, most of the literature on grief and mourning concentrates on personal and social experiences of bereavement surrounding death. But increasing attention is being paid to grief and mourning over other types of loss ranging from divorce to disfigurement. See Gregory Rochlin, *Griefs and Discontents, The Forces of Change* (Boston: Little, Brown and Company, 1965); *Loss and Grief: Psychological Management in Medical Practice*, ed. by Bernard Schoenberg, Arthur C. Carr, David Peretz, and Austin H. Kutscher (New York: Columbia University Press, 1970), pp. 119–220; Parkes, *Bereavement*, pp. 200–213.

14. Kliever, "Dax and Job: The Refusal of Redemptive Suffering," in *Dax's Case*, pp. 187–221. Contrary to what some of my readers have charged, my purpose in comparing Dax to Job was not to chide Dax for not availing himself of any Judeo-Christian responses

to suffering as redemptive. Rather, I was suggesting to Dax that there are positive religious and philosophical responses to suffering (both ancient and modern) which do not "explain away" suffering by crediting suffering itself for achieving some higher purpose or larger good.

15. This is the point that William F. May makes in the chapter on "The Burned" in his book, *The Patient's Ordeal* (Bloomington: Indiana University Press, 1991), pp. 15–35. May shows that repairing damaged bodies is not the same thing as restoring shattered lives. Catastrophic illnesses shatter old identities, leaving the victim ill-prepared to go on living. Forging a new identity is a task of reconstruction and rebirth.

16. Dax has participated in an Anthony Robbins "Firewalking Seminar." See Anthony Robbins, *Unlimited Power* (New York: Fawcett Columbine, 1986).

17. William Steele, *Cornell Alumni News* (February 1983), 22–25; John Lee Smith, *Cornell Law Forum*, Vol. 9 (1983): 15–18.

18. David B. Morris, *The Culture of Pain* (Berkeley: University of California Press, 1991), p. 9.

19. Ibid., p. 3.

20. Peter L. Berger, *The Sacred Canopy, Elements of a Sociological Theory of Religion* (New York: Doubleday & Co., 1969), pp. 54–55.

21. Jay Katz, *The Silent World of Doctor and Patient* (New York: The Free Press, 1984), pp. 1–29.

22. Ibid., pp. 226–227.

23. Richard M. Zaner, "Failed Or On-Going Dialogues? Dax's Case," in *Dax's Case*, Kliever (ed.), pp. 43–61.

24. For explorations of chronic illness and permanent disability from the patient's and family's viewpoint, see Arthur Kleinman, *The Illness Narrative, Suffering, Healing, and the Human Condition* (New York: Basic Books, Inc., 1988); William F. May, *The Patient's Ordeal.* For illness narratives drawn from literature, see Howard Brody, *Stories of Sickness* (New Haven: Yale University Press, 1987). For autobiographical accounts of illness, see Arthur W. Frank, *At the Will of the Body, Reflections on Illness* (Boston: Houghton Mifflin Company, 1991); Terry Pringle, *This Is the Boy* (Dallas: Southern Methodist University Press, 1992).

5

WHOSE STORY IS IT ANYWAY?

Authority, Voice, and Responsibility in Narratives of Chronic Illness

SUE E. ESTROFF

Introduction

There is a kind of cold, quiet terror that comes with a telephone ring at 3 A.M. Almost always, there is something to hear that one would rather not. And so it was that night—the confusion of sleep vanished in a second, replaced by nausea borne of fear. The voice I heard was almost chanting in rage and anguish. There was ridicule, too, and precision cuts at my fast-fading concepts of myself as a kind, careful, and just ethnographer. She had asked for a copy of the book I had written about her and the others. I gave it to her as a gift. She had just read what I had written about her ten years before. She was wounded by the images of herself in the past—psychotic, rambling, wise, and charming. I had exploited her, used her, misunderstood everything, and was unmasked now, she said. Not the bright, "liberal," sympathetic researcher I claimed to be, but worse than the others for my self- and other deception. Furthered my career, made a name for myself, all at her expense. How could you? (By now I was asking this silently, along with her.) How could you come see me again, spend the whole day with me, like a friend, pretending to understand, to like me?

The facts were not in dispute—their public presence and meaning, and my commentary were. Seeing the now non-sensical notes she wrote when psychotic, seeing herself at that bewildered time on the printed page were somehow intolerable. She chanted on in howling pain and anger; nothing I said made any difference. I was shaking by now, desperate to intervene, to break the grip of the agony now swallowing both of us. Could we meet and talk it over? No. I never want to talk to you again. Could I please explain what I had written, place it in the broader context of the book? Had she read the rest of it? No. No. Was there anything I could say or do to help? No. Please, would she accept my apology? No. She hung up. I called back. Don't ever bother me again. I apologized once more. She hung up again.

EVEN THOUGH THIS incident took place over seven years ago, I am haunted still by this woman's voice, by the penetrating pain that I caused, and by the perplexing questions raised by this episode and other, far less dramatic and far more positive exchanges with informants over the years. I was never able to determine exactly what I had written about her that was so disturbing to her. Should this woman have had editorial veto authority (Capron 1991) over the text before publication? How tempting it was (and is) to view her response as an "overreaction," as a symptom of her psychiatric problems (and the self-described abrupt tirades that left her few friends, even fewer restaurants where she was welcome), instead of a legitimate cry of foul and indignation. What responsibilities did I have to protect her from the pain of recognizing herself in a prior state that later humiliated and undermined her well-being? It is a story about her, but my account is privileged. She has no access to a comparable forum in which to dispute or respond to my representation of her (except perhaps here, and still I intervene). Should I even be telling *this* story?

My intention in this interrogative essay is to articulate some of the important but "unsung" (Barnard 1985) tensions and ethical dilemmas generated in the production of knowledge about persons with chronic illness, particularly in the production of chronic illness narrative research. In my view, when we engage in this work, there is an underlying potential for conflict between the demands of scholarly inquiry for accuracy, authenticity, and disclosure, and the demands of professional ethics and interpersonal morality for the protection, if not enhancement, of individual dignity, autonomy, privacy, and well-being (see also Davis 1991). As we engage in qualitative, profoundly subject-centered research on chronic illness and call for increasing attention to the biographical, experiencing person, ironically we may simultaneously raise the ethical stakes and multiply the potential for compromising those principles which we bring and which bring us to the subject at the outset. When we convey this rich totality we may also unmask the person, reveal secrets, uncover hidden hopes and fears—to an audience of strangers, and sometimes to the person as well (see King & Stanford 1992). How do we formulate and respond to these challenges? What is the nature and extent of our responsibility to the persons whose lives we learn from and write about, during and after the research process?

There are some characteristics of the chronic illness experience, and of people with enduring disablements, that complicate these questions and make responding to them vital. These include the presence and importance of Others (caregivers, relatives, friends) and Institutions (hospitals, agencies); the duration of the research relationship and the disabling condition; the processes of protest, denial, acceptance, reformulation, and resignation that prevail in varying sequences in our informants' lives; their quasi sociopolitical status as a protected but nonetheless marginalized, stigmatized group; and their substantial poverty, and their financial and instrumental dependence on familial and social resources. The illness narrative research process takes place within and influences this intricate weave of persons, experiences, and conditions.

These questions are also of particular relevance in the domain of chronic illness because of our obligation, as clinicians and researchers, to assist in "sustaining an intact, well-integrated self who is in control of, not controlled by the illness" (Jennings, Callahan, & Caplan 1988:11). The recent Hastings Center gathering on the ethical challenges of chronic illness did not address research explicitly (an interesting omission), and concluded that "The primary obligation of chronic care medicine, then, is . . . to assist the person in keeping the transformative power of illness under control, to integrate new subjective interests (wants) and new objective interests (needs) into a coherent and satisfying life" (ibid.). Leaving aside the differing obligations and roles of clinicians and researchers (see Churchill 1980), the question becomes whether or how the research relationship, process, and product may promote, impede, or even reverse this process.

If chronic illness represents an inevitable loss of authority, control, and self, do we in some way replicate or worsen this process by our intense focus on illness-related experience, compounded by the narrative privilege of the author/scholar? Or do we perhaps reverse and counteract the sense of loss and isolation by giving some additional voice and empathic moments of reflection to the subject that they would not otherwise have? Both of these possibilities pertain in the case of one study participant:

> [from interviewer notes] A. found the SASB [a psychological scale] very upsetting and stated toward the end that she felt very shaky. She did say that she would continue and so we finished it. Afterward she said, "I physically don't feel good. That made me feel very ill." She needed to talk for quite a while afterward before she felt more calm. . . . The SASB stirred strong feelings of anger toward her parents. She feels she is manic to escape her parents, that they are suffocating her. At the end of the entire interview she stated, "This study is an inspiration to me to be more honest and open with my therapist too."

I do not aim here (because I am unable) to answer this heap of questions or to propose solutions to these dilemmas. Nor have I set out to review comprehensively prior thinking on germane subjects such as informed consent, moral agency, authorial signature, and current debate and practice in ethnography (Comaroff &

Comaroff 1991; Geertz 1988; Personal Narratives Group 1989). The idea is to vocalize, frame, and further the discussion for a relatively narrow purpose and audience.

The primary data are my work of nearly two decades with one group of individuals with severe, persistent mental illnesses (Estroff 1985), and the interview texts, experiences, and commentary of my research team over the past six years with another, larger group of similar people. I have drawn also (and pragmatically) on rather disparate bodies of thought and practice—bioethics, interpretative and postmodernist ethnography and ethnographic commentary, feminist criticism, oral history, illness narratives, and social research ethics. Equal measures of comfort and despair come from the surmise that most of the questions raised here are not new and that many minds with diverse perspectives are grappling with similar concerns. While there is some consensus about the dilemmas, none of us has imagined or invented satisfactory solutions. This essay is neither a postmodernist's self-critical, deconstructive wail nor a positivist's rationale or apology (see Johannsen 1992; Patai 1991). In some ways, this is a narrative of the illness narrative process, an ethnographic sketch of the work of illness ethnography.

The domains of authority, voice, and responsibility—personal and academic, of the subject and of the scholar—seem to be central to these concerns and are the focus of this initial query. Authority refers to the special access to resources, audience, and the legitimated construction of knowledge that comes with academic and clinical credentials, publications, and funded research. Authority also derives from experience, from unique or extraordinary knowledge, and resides in those who know what we wish to discover and understand—this is the authority of the subject. Voice has to do with words and thoughts, speech that is usually transformed into text, with the style, texture, nuance, and shape of the story and the narrative. My authorial voice is reflected in my choice of metaphor, analogy, adjective, and what I say (and do not) both in the interview and in the resultant text. The voices of informants are on tape, in my head, and eventually on the page—conveyed as fragile cargo or as blaring message. Responsibility concerns conduct with regard to the Other: how I work with informants—how I participate in the consent process; conduct the interview; spend time with subjects; work with data; present ideas and findings; and respond to the consequences of those findings. The responsibilities of informants are less apparent, but include communication of their comforts and discomforts, their concerns about and agendas for the relationship between us, and some consideration for the privacy and sensibilities of their Others.

In this paper, I explore authority, voice, and responsibility in scholar-subject or researcher-informant relations. The topics of scholar-scholar relations and the triangle of scholar-subject-other (the subject's others) relations are equally important, but are in the background here.

Situating the Problems and the Discourse

We engage in this reflection at a particular historical moment characterized by two forces of special relevance:[1] commodification—particularly of ideas, stories, and words; and patient/consumer self-advocacy and activism.

Commodifying Voice and Experience

The title of this essay[2] conveys the possibility of ownership of the story, indeed, implies a proprietorship of the self-of-the-story as an entity, over which an individual exercises authority. This is sometimes referred to in the field of ethics as autonomy. While autonomy and moral agency are principles easily endorsed, the ensuing commodification of a narrative as the "property" of this agent or that researcher causes some discomfort.

The production of illness narratives is at best an explicitly collaborative effort (Brody 1987; Frank 1979, 1988; Liebow 1993), yet there is wide latitude in the ability and interest of our informants to participate as collaborators. Some of the people I work with express interest in what will become of their interview responses and our conversations. The following interview excerpt illustrates how we respond to these queries (I=interviewer, R=respondent):

I: That's real helpful. Anything that you want to tell me about, or that's happened, or that you think about that I haven't asked you about?

R: Not really. Except if I ask you what you're going to do with all that.

I: Well, I'm going to put it together with—there are about 170 people [in the study].

R: Wow, that many Sue?

I: Like you, and that we're trying to learn from. There are four other people that work with me, that know people like you, and who see them every six months the same way I see you—and that care about them, and get to know them, and sit down and have conversations like this. And then we try to put that all together and see if there are any patterns. If there are things that people say, more than one person says, that will teach us better how to be there for people like you that are trying to make a life for themselves. And so we can understand, not what's in the textbooks and [what] the other doctors say, but what your experience is.

R: Yeah, like A. [job coach] said to me. She said, Would I feel better dropping this job and having us find something else? And the truth inside me is, I'd rather not be pushed like this. But I couldn't say it to her, so I just said, "No," because it is a job and it's there.

I: My goal really is to understand your experience and your, if you will, truth. Because I think that's more important than laboratories and tests and stuff like that.

R: Because you get yourself all prepared for a laboratory, don't you?

I: Yeah. And the way that you tell me, and the way that I learn from you is really more helpful. And hopefully, if we put this all together and make some sense of it, we can come back to the people here at the mental health center and say, totally honestly, that these 170 people we talked to all this time, and got to know, and to care about, told us that this is what their lives were like. And that this would help and that would help. And maybe not what you're [the mental health center] doing here, but something else.

R: Oh, I see. That sounds nice, Sue.

The message is collaborative: what you say will help us to make the mental health system better—we will convey your voice, your experience to others. This person, like several others, responded by contrasting the "truth" of what she told us with what she told treatment personnel, reinforcing the "trusted messenger" role that we claimed. Yet there is no claim, no glimmer, of ownership of the message from her. Ironically, I gain authority as a researcher, as a would-be-reformer of mental health services, by invoking her authority and by telling her story, which has by now become my consultation, my report, my article.

Most informants, however, do not ask about what form their words will take eventually; they are concerned mainly with confidentiality—that what they say will not be conveyed to people they know, particularly mental health professionals or their families. Their concerns revolve around their recognition by known others. Self-recognition—the wound of the person described at the beginning of this essay—has never since been voiced. Our consent form states explicitly that there will be publications based on the data. No one in the current study has asked to see what we produce. Yet I doubt seriously that the woman whose words are reproduced above ever imagined that they would appear in a paper like this, or would be read/heard by strangers. Would she feel differently about her participation if I sent her a copy of this paper? What canons of consent and collaboration would dictate that I do so?

I suspect that one reason so few informants express any sort of ownership or ask for research results is because they associate us and our study with the medical / institutional establishment, and therefore confer on us a type of privilege by proxy. The most common sort of illness narrative or biography consists of the medical chart and the clinicians's notes, which have historically *belonged* to the physician and the institution (hospital or clinic) wherein treatment occurs. Clinicians traditionally have had the unchallenged authority to create and control access to the official text of the illness experience (see Barrett 1988; Stoller 1988). Likewise, ethnographers have viewed their field notes, tapes, and transcripts as quasi-sacred, as *theirs.*

Reconstruing the chart as a type of illness narrative (or pre-narrative) produced in collaboration (however uneasy or implicit), and therefore as a shared product, turns this authority on its head. While patients have the right to read their charts, very few are aware of this or do, and they are barred from the act of inscription in them. Similarly, except in the most experimental of ethnographies, informants do not write the text, though they may provide journals or written materials to the researcher. Both ethnographer and clinician have claimed the right of privacy for their thoughts and interpretations in charts and field notes, also expressing some concern about the potential harm to the patient/informant should the unspoken observation or diagnosis be revealed to them. It is within these traditions that the question of "whose story" is nested.

Something important happens in the transformation from conversation to interview, and from spoken word to published text (Patai 1991). When the chart provides the data for a published case study, or the fieldnotes or tapes provide the informant's voice for a published article, the rules and nature of the problem change. At this juncture, there is another audience and a different purpose for the text, the ownership and authority of the author is established, and the commodification process is actual and irreversible.[3]

One long-standing solution to the appropriation by clinicians or ethnographers of the stories of persons who are ill, and to the perceived mistranslations that appear in academic discourse, is the autobiographical or first-person illness account (e.g., Murphy 1989; Peterson 1982; Styron 1990; Jeffries et al. 1990; Zola 1982). In this genre, the person speaks for and of herself, often, but not always, because of or in response to other or competing versions of the story (see especially Chamberlin 1978; Vonnegut 1975). Whether and how illness narrative—and the continuum from information (charts, interviews, transcripts) to knowledge (texts, published articles)—are commodities, and whose, are problems that must be addressed.[4]

Advocacy and Activism: Consumer Counterclaims

At the same time, and not coincidentally, patient/consumer advocacy and activism in political, clinical, and research arenas by persons with chronic illnesses and disabilities are more robust and widespread than at any previous time. In the psychiatric area, current and former patients are engaged in unprecedented activities—serving on journal editorial boards, conducting research, participating in scientific meetings, running their own treatment programs, demanding and often having an influence on policy decisions and a voice in public debate about their care and treatment. Self-help groups with a variety of goals are flourishing all over the globe. Every area of professional authority is being contested—from involuntary commitment to the allocation of public mental health dollars.

To complicate matters further, we encounter the other Other—the caregiver, relative, and significant other of the person with a chronic, disabling condition. Like physicians and ethnographers, these others have until recently spoken unchallenged for and about their loved ones with disabilities. The National Alliance for the Mentally Ill, a group of parents and relatives of persons with mental illnesses (they now call them neurobiological disorders, or NBD), has become the most powerful lobby promoting biological psychiatric research, expansion of mental health resources at the federal, state, and local level, and a profoundly disease-based conception of mental illness (McLean 1990). This collective Other voice is sometimes quite dissonant with the stated desires of consumers—and a struggle for authority to voice and define those wishes and needs is underway.

The voices of psychiatric consumers remain largely spoken—at meetings and conferences where they may tell their own stories in a kind of confessional or witnessing mode, or where they challenge professionals who are speaking *about* them. How well I recall the voice of a prominent consumer leader booming from the back of a crowded lecture hall where I had just spoken with some urgency about consumer rights and voice: "If you believe all that stuff you just said, then how come you're up there instead of me?" There are comparable developments among persons with AIDS and among a variety of groups formed around particular disabling conditions. This assertion of authority and sounding of voice requires a serious scholarly response as well as a political one[5] (see Campbell 1991; Estroff & Strauss 1989; Zola 1991).

Ways of Knowing about Persons with Chronic Illness: What We Say and Do

What We Say about Authority, Voice, and Responsibility

In his introduction to Paul Rabinow's *Reflections on Fieldwork in Morocco* (1977), Robert Bellah asserts that "knowing in the human studies is always emotional and moral as well as intellectual" (xi). This is by now an almost commonplace "truth" among us, but the meaning of this position with special reference to the ways that we "know" about illness, particularly persons with chronic illnesses, remains to be made explicit. What does "emotional and moral knowing" mean in practice? Now that the objectivist jig is up and the truth is out (in more ways than one), it seems that matters are more cloudy and charged—anything but clearer. As Geertz (1988:130–131) observes wryly,

> The gap between engaging others where they are and representing them where they aren't, always immense but not much noticed, has suddenly become extremely visible. What once seemed only technically difficult, getting "their" lives into "our" works, has turned morally, politically, even epistemologically, delicate. . . . What is at hand is a pervasive nervousness about the whole business of claiming to explain enigmatical others on the grounds that you have gone about with them in their native habitat. . . .

A frankly opportunistic review of approaches to these quandaries yielded several (crude and overlapping) types of practice and position.[6] These are:

1. Conceptual and theoretical (Marcus & Fischer 1986; Comaroff & Comaroff 1991; Geertz 1973, 1988; Jackson 1989);
2. Ideological and political (Fine & Asch 1988; Personal Narratives Group 1989; Patai 1991; Conquergood 1991, 1992; Dula 1991);
3. Psychological and Psychoanalytic (Crapanzano 1980);
4. Personal/journal-istic (Rabinow 1977; Lévi-Strauss 1967; Zola 1982);
5. Clinical (Kleinman 1988; Brody 1987; Strauss 1989);
6. Philosophical/ethical and legal/ethical (Churchill & Churchill 1982;

Churchill 1980; Brody 1987; Gostin 1991; Dickens, Gostin & Levine 1991; McCarthy & Porter 1991; Marshall 1992).

These works abound with elegant elucidation of the conceptual allure of phenomenology, subjectivity, and reflexivity, of relational knowledge as the fulcrum of our work, and of the intellectual arrogance and hegemony we carry with us inexorably to the field or clinic. The ethical and legal views take us deeply into the meanings of autonomy, consent, harms as different from wrongs, and the rule of torts and privacy. However satisfying intellectually and inspiring ideologically, there is little here that satisfies the moral, interpersonal, and ethical quandaries of the actual research act and process, and their consequences. To put it baldly, nearly everyone identifies and decries the same problems, albeit with different vocabularies and agendas, but few of us seem to actually *do* or *produce the work* much differently (see Conquergood 1992; Personal Narratives Group 1989; and Reinharz 1992 for some exceptions).

Despite the "pervasive nervousness," ethical language and principles have seldom been invoked or applied explicitly to the production of knowledge in the ethnographic and qualitative study of illness. Focusing narrowly on qualitative chronic illness narrative research, my equally idiosyncratic review revealed a near total absence of discussion of ethical or moral dilemmas raised in and by the research process. Gelya Frank (1979) and Robert Stoller (1988) are perhaps the most explicit in this regard, but their collaborations are exceptions. Stoller, for example, engages in a process whereby "patients know they will see each version [of an article about them] and can modify and delete, even on galleys" (1988:373). Nearly all of the material related to confidentiality, to the research relationship, and to the production of the narrative was in the footnotes, preface, or acknowledgments. Consent, privacy, self- (as opposed to other) recognition as a consideration, and other basic ethical principles of the research were rarely mentioned. Most of us express deep gratitude to and admiration for our informants, but go no further. Even the most intensely personal and revealing narratives are presented without any mention of the role of or agreements made with the subject (see for example Ratey, Sands, & Driscoll 1986; Crapanzano 1980; Bouricius 1989). Typically, there was a statement that the subject's identity was being disguised in various ways (usually a pseudonym), and a warning that some potentially identifying features had been altered (see for example Kleinman 1988:33, note 1).

Conrad's (1987) review of research on chronic illness experience reminds the reader that patients are really people, yet goes no further in the section on meth-

odological problems. Charmaz's (1983, 1987) exceptionally thoughtful and elo-
quent articulations of the loss of and struggle for self in chronic illness acknowledge the contributions of professional colleagues. Ironically there is no exposition
of the role of informants or of the research relationship and process in the text.

In my view, this amounts to an absence of methodological as well as moral
rigor. Relegating this discourse (literally) to the margins of our work seems to me
a shortcoming. At the same time, I am not suggesting that process tyrannize content, or that we overtake the richness of the narrative with agonized apologies for
appropriating someone's story.

What guidelines should then be followed when seeking to know and then communicate about the other who is ill—perhaps compromised, vulnerable, searching
for answers to technical and existential questions, seeking to make sense of a complicated, intimate process? I find this especially problematic because I work primarily with persons who have psychiatric disorders of a severe and prolonged nature. Some of the people I work with do not believe, or dread deeply, that they
have a mental illness. They go to great lengths to persuade me that they are not
mentally ill, and to elicit my corroboration of their views. One treads carefully
here, especially when a casual remark or a moment's lapse, or the interview itself,
indicates that I think otherwise (see Estroff et al. 1991). Their private terrors and
wisdom, along with their public conduct, are the data of my research. Many of
them are exquisitely sensitive to invasions of privacy, being misunderstood, and
being stigmatized—their perceptions pathologized or discounted by others. These
are valid concerns, and trust is constructed carefully, slowly. The accompanying
responsibilities I incur to honor that trust and respond to these concerns are what
concern us here.

I examined the codes of ethics for anthropologists, psychiatrists, and psychologists, the most relevant professions for the people with whom I work, in search of
prescriptions and proscriptions related to the questions raised. Many of the ethical principles for scholarly conduct with "human subjects" are either so ambiguous and broad as to defy operationalization, or so specific to clinical interventions
and laboratory settings as to be irrelevant to illness narrative research. Each code
has the unmistakable signs of being produced by a committee, rife with bold assertions accompanied by disclaimers, and are internally contradictory in some
cases. For example, the obligation to make clear to informants that one really cannot safeguard their anonymity in all cases seems contradictory with the idea that
when conflicts arise, the informants' interests come first. Each code also fails in
varying degrees to define the nature and meaning of anonymity and to address
whose measure of respect for dignity and privacy should prevail. It is my unhappy

assessment that despite these deficits, these ethical principles, followed to the letter and in intent, would preclude or radically alter much of the chronic illness narrative work that we have done. For example, were I to discontinue work, as the anthropological code says I should, each time I anticipated a potentially negative consequence for someone who might read what I have written, I could write precious little. Safeguarding the sensitivities of informants is not always compatible with relating events and utterances as they occur—as with the person I described at the beginning of this essay.

The statement of ethics of the American Anthropological Association (AAA 1990) asserts that:

> Anthropologists' first responsibility is to those whose lives and cultures they study. Should conflicts arise, the interests of these people take precedence over other considerations. . . . The rights, interests, safety, and sensitivities of those who entrust information to anthropologists must be safeguarded. The right of those providing information to anthropologists either to remain anonymous or to receive recognition is to be respected and defended. It is the responsibility of anthropologists to make every effort to determine the preferences of those providing information and to comply with those wishes. It should be made clear to anyone providing information that despite the anthropologist's best intentions and efforts anonymity may be compromised or recognition fail to materialize. . . . Anthropologists have an ongoing obligation to assess both the positive and negative consequences of their activities and the publications resulting from those activities. . . . *If they anticipate the possibility that such violations [of professional responsibility] might occur, they should take steps, including, if necessary, discontinuance of work, to avoid such outcomes.* (italics in original, underlining mine)

Was the unintentional yet undeniable damage done to the well-being of my former informant a violation of these principles and of nonmaleficence? The informant's interests were unarticulated, and became clear and in conflict only after the narrative was produced and published. Was it my responsibility to make certain that she could not be harmed and offended, to anticipate that she might? Would this paralyze my research and writing, or am I making the same old claim to the privilege and authority of the scholar by suggesting so?

On the matters at hand, the psychiatrists also promulgate noble enough principles, and are predictably more explicit about the special considerations that obtain when working with patients. For example:

> The psychiatrist should diligently guard against exploiting information furnished by the patient, and should not use the unique position of power afforded him/her by the psychotherapeutic situation to influence the patient in any way not directly relevant to treatment goals. . . . Clinical and other materials used in teaching and

writing must be <u>adequately disguised in order to preserve the anonymity of the individuals involved</u>. . . . With regard for the <u>dignity and privacy</u> and with <u>truly informed consent</u>, it is ethical to <u>present a patient</u> to a scientific gathering, if the confidentiality of the presentation is understood and accepted by the <u>audience</u>. . . . When involved in funded research, the ethical psychiatrist will advise human subjects of the funding source, <u>retain his/her freedom to reveal data and results</u>, and follow all appropriate and current guidelines relative to human subject protection. (American Psychiatric Association 1986) (emphasis mine)

The psychologists take a comparable stance, but are much more explicit about the conduct of research per se:

[Psychologists should] plan their research in ways to minimize the possibility that their <u>findings will be mis-leading</u>. . . . In publishing reports of their work, <u>they never suppress disconfirming data</u>. . . . the psychologist carries out the investigation with respect and concern for the dignity and welfare of the people who participate. . . . Where research procedures result in <u>undesirable consequences for the individual participant, the investigator has the responsibility to detect and remove or correct these consequences, including long-term effects</u>. Information obtained about a research participant during the course of an investigation is confidential unless otherwise agreed in advance. When the possibility exists that others may obtain access to such information, this possibility, together with the plans for protecting confidentiality, is explained to the participant as part of the procedure for obtaining informed consent. (American Psychological Association 1989) (emphasis mine)

Each of us exploits unavoidably—our careers and stature advance with each publication about an informant, but do their circumstances or esteem increase comparably, or at all? We cannot protect the privacy and preferences of participants if we never suppress disconfirming information. Freedom to reveal data cannot be absolute. How can we adequately disguise identity—who decides what is an adequate disguise?—without being misleading in some way? (Davis 1991). These and many more gaps between principle and practice arise, and deserve some attention and debate.

What We Do about Authority, Voice, and Responsibility

In the awesome shadow/harsh light of these ethical principles, and with some trepidation, I describe some of the dilemmas that have arisen in our current research, and how we have attempted to resolve conflicting interests and moral quandaries. We have come to the view that consent is an ongoing process—never completed and seldom "truly informed," but a helpful framework and goal to keep always in mind. Consent and collaboration are negotiated in ongoing, complicated relationships with our informants, relationships which sometimes generate conflicts with our tasks and roles as researchers. We consider responding to these challenges to be as important a part of the research process as the data we collect and the analyses we conduct.

In order to monitor and examine the research process, every interviewer dictated notes *about* the interview, and their experiences and impressions, each time they interacted with an informant. The highlight of our regular project meetings was what we called storytelling—extensive and free-flowing accounts of interviews conducted that week, including discussion of how and what the informant was doing, what the impact of the visit and interview were, and questions about how far to pursue a reluctant or evasive participant, and the like. We often learned as much for analysis purposes from the interviewer's narrative as we did from the interview forms. As importantly, we developed a collective process for coming to terms with dilemmas that confronted us in our relationships with the participants, and in meeting the demands of the study—in view of those relationships.

Life Course, Illness Course. Longitudinal research with persons engaged in a longitudinal illness experience, especially one that is so disruptive of person, relations, and psyche, is influenced by countless, often uncontrollable factors. For example, when we happen to encounter the person, and where, changes what we learn. As one informant observed wisely:

> I think I feel better now. I think if you interview me—it's funny you know, you talk about interviewing people with mental illness, you know. Initially I was interviewed in the hospital, so I'm in a different environment. I think these things affect, or should affect the study. And I then, I have sometimes real bad days. I know I've been interviewed on a bad day. I was interviewed after my house burned down. (chuckle) You've got different influences going on here. I think today is a good time. I think what I'm saying is pretty accurate. And I think probably some of what I've said in the past was accurate. But, on a day when I feel better I can give you a more accurate picture.

We had an interview schedule to meet, and an ever-present concern over missing interviews and losing participants. Many a time we rescheduled, broke the interview into small sessions, or adapted the format in various ways to accommodate the needs and abilities of the participants. To illustrate:

> [interviewer notes] Within the first few pages of the interview, B. S. demonstrated that he was having some difficulties in that he was shaking. He brought this under control and within a few more pages began to rock steadily. . . . At page 67, he asked for a break, but returned once again very quickly. At page 72 he began to

tremble so violently that although he insisted that he wanted to finish the interview, we were finally forced to stop. When I returned again in a few days time, he was eager to complete the interview. He said that he found it very embarrassing to be unable to control his shaking and that he felt that was due to problems of medication.

The psychiatric condition of the participants varied from interview to interview, and even within one session. The skill, persistence, and sometimes courage of our team were called on repeatedly. For example:

[interviewer notes] . . . he became sort of suspicious of my motives with the survey and called his therapist and tried to verify that indeed, the Triangle Mental Health Survey is a valid organ of the University. He did contact the doctor's wife and she sort of rummaged around, found some forms we'd sent him [to obtain his consent to contact his therapist, and to give permission to the therapist to release to us the number of his visits], and said, 'Yes,' so he felt better. . . . in the process of trying to determine this, F. came up to me and grabbed my hand very tightly and put his face right up next to mine, and in a very pressured voice and angry tone said, "I've got to find out about this because my brother's in the CIA, and they'll use me to get to him." And then right after that, as soon as he realized what he had been saying, he stopped and apologized and said, "No, I'm sorry. Let's stop and shake hands the way we're supposed to." And that was sort of the pattern for the interview. Other interesting features of the interview included F.'s tendency to use the bathroom. He did it about 15 times in a period of 2 1/2 hours. . . . He would not close the door, and would just kind of stand and over his shoulder say, "It's O.K., go ahead. Next question." So, I'd ask the question, and he'd yell a response back to me, "very often" [from a symptom scale], or whatever the answer may be.

Who Are We Anyway? Ambiguity, Affection, and Role. The lines between friend and investigator blur over time, producing almost as many difficulties as positive contributions to the quality of the research. Identifying who we were—both to others and in their lives—resulted in a variety of responses by the participants. One woman introduced me to her father as "her doctor," but when I went to choir practice with her at her all-black church, she introduced me as a friend. Several men told fellow patients that the interviewer was their "girl friend," and some inquired as to establishing such a relationship.

These ambiguous relationships led to some perplexing problems, especially over the nearly three years of association. There was intimacy and then absence; there was deeply personal revelation and then the payment of a subject fee—sometimes refused because it offended the intimacy, a blunt reminder that there was a purpose for the intimacy that seemed cold and pragmatic. At other times respondents refused the payment because they benefitted from and enjoyed their contact with us. For example, [interviewer notes] " . . . he was the only person who has refused to accept the money. No matter what I said to him about trying to give him the money, he would not take it. And I said that, you know, he was doing us a big favor. His response was, 'You all are doing me a big favor.' " Another participant said in response to the question Has anything good happened lately? "Well, you coming here is something good." One person asked, "Why can't *you* be my doctor?" And still another contrasted the quality of our relationship with the one she had with her case managers:

I: So what would be helpful for you that you aren't getting?

R: Probably if I had been left here, you know, for all the time I've been here, and somebody had just talked to me like you did, rather than going through all these other things and hiding it all. . . .

I: So somebody really to be with you and talk with you, and someone you trusted and who liked you.

R: Yeah, if they were there like that, rather than talking, you know, so spacey and all that stuff like that. Then having to agree with it in order to get along with it and cope with it.

I: Who talks spacey? They talk spacey or you talk spacey?

R: They talk spacey to me. Because like they say, "when you get your own place" and like that. You know what I mean. It's like it goes in one ear and out the other. . . . That's bullshit talk.

I: So, less bullshit would be helpful. One person that's kind of there for you.

R: Yeah, like you talk to me. . . . if I think of what would be helpful to me, then I'd say, well, let's start this whole thing over and forget this nonsense that we've been doing in the past . . . and let's be friends, or you know, like you and I are.

Each of us developed varying degrees of attachment to the people we learned from, and struggled to come to a comfortable position in this regard. There was no rule about being "too involved," and amount and type of involvement was discussed openly in our meetings.

The informants' views of themselves and us, and the research we were engaged in, changed, sometimes radically, over time. While at one interview I might be seen as an empathic and trusted other, at another I was a disquieting intrusion. One of the people I followed in the study literally ran into her house and locked the door when she saw me coming for our fourth interview. Since she had no telephone, I had left several notes which were unanswered, and had no inkling of her desire to avoid me. At a later interview she apologized profusely saying, "I was a mess. I didn't want you to see me that way, but I didn't know how to tell you. Well, I wanted to talk to you, but I didn't want to do that interview."

Obligation, Remuneration, and Participation. Several times now, the apology of a study participant to an interviewer has been reported, and this deserves some comment, along with the subject of money. We found that many informants took their consent to participate in the study quite seriously, considering it almost an obligation. Each agreed to the two-year follow-up in the initial consent discussion, and was aware that we would contact them at six-month intervals. Despite explicit provisions for withdrawal from the study, which were underscored in this process, some of them were clearly reluctant to do so because of this sense of obligation, because of their relationships with us, and because many needed the money. Only three actually withdrew from the study, though some others may have accomplished the same ends by avoiding us or not responding to contact letters or phone calls. Two of those who withdrew did so because participation was intolerable to them as a labeling experience. They did not consider themselves to be mentally ill, and the interview and its content were too powerful a disconfirmation.

Many of these elements are illustrated in the following excerpt:

[interviewer notes] T. has asked to be let out of the study . . . he said he did not want to do anymore interviews. This came rather suddenly. He had called me, once again responding to a letter, and seemed really hot to do the interview. I think he needed the money. . . . during the interview itself, he made comments such as he didn't like a lot of the questions we asked because they presupposed that he was mentally ill. He did not like that supposition. This was particularly tough on some of the questions, for example the PERI Scale [psychiatric symptoms]. . . . He asked me how many more [interviews] we would be doing, how many were left, and I said there would be two more. He said, Gosh, did he really have to do it? That he was "fed up" with doing it. . . . He said, "I'm telling you now that I don't want to do it. Can't I just stop now?" And I said, "Well, if that's the way you really feel about it, sure you can." And so, "That's the way I feel about it," he said.

"Do I really have to do it" and "can't I just stop now" make very clear the sense of obligation to continue and the difficulty of quitting that were a product of the consent, the relationship, and the idea that the interviews were somehow a test or a measure of ability. We tried to avoid replicating in ourselves the sense of failing an obligation when an interview was missed or someone withdrew. At the same time, we had to weigh carefully the need to complete as many interviews as possible against the fluctuating preferences, condition, and circumstances of the participants.

Is Probing Giving Voice? As is already apparent, the interview was sometimes salve and sometimes salt, sometimes both at once. To illustrate:

[interviewer notes] M. got very upset in doing the Time 4 interview. When we got to page 15 just after the employment section, she burst out, "This interview is making me pissy. I wonder why. It's very personal." We went on to talk again about the aims of the study and the purpose of the questions. M. stated, "If some of the doctors there [at the University hospital] don't change their attitude, I don't know what's going to happen. They really do not care. They thought they were superior to me and to the other patients. They have an incredible arrogant attitude." After discussing these feelings for a brief amount of time, M. agreed to continue the interview. At the end, she even apologized indirectly.

[interviewer notes] Just after the very first questions of the social support section, when S. mentioned her mother and father, she suddenly and very surprisingly burst into tears, crying in an almost hysterical manner. When asked what was wrong, she said, "I miss my family." With sympathy and calm reassurance she stopped crying, dried her eyes, and went on as though nothing had happened.

In the first instance, the informant was able to voice her concerns about how the doctors had treated her, but she felt bad about her employment failures and clearly experienced the interview as intrusive and upsetting. In the second case, we tread on sore ground, with less obvious benefit to or reciprocal exchange with the respondent.

Voice and Audience. One aspect of voice that concerned us was truth-telling, disclosure, and revealing secrets. We invited, probably expected, our informants to disclose to us. Yet we withheld opinions, information, and observations from them, particularly when asked if we thought they were mentally ill, if the doctor's diagnosis was correct, or when what they told us was in direct conflict with information we had from other sources (especially charts). In essence, our voices were carefully, purposefully controlled, while we hoped that those of the informants were not. No doubt, some participants monitored themselves similarly. As one woman said after an interview, and when her friend approached, "Now, let's get down to some real talking."

In the interview the informant's voice predominates, while mine is muted and in the background. In the text my voice sounds much different—but seldom do informants hear/read that voice. I hear their voices, but they rarely hear mine. In this sense, we privilege another audience with a voice of privilege. In the live interview, I avoid the claim of a voice of authority. When I create the text, I take that authority. However wise or necessary this selective disclosure and my differing voices may be, collaboration and reciprocity with informants are inevitably reduced, if not undermined.

At the same time, it seems especially important to regulate our voices because of the delicate processes of sense-making and self-assessing that our informants are engaged in. We sought to observe and understand rather than to direct or influence these projects. Nearly everyone else in our informants' lives commented on, judged, assessed, or defined them—how they were, what was wrong, what they should do. We deliberately took a place apart from these others. While we took this posture for methodological reasons, it has been apparent to us that a non-judgemental, (even if only occasionally) unconditionally interested, listening other was usually quite welcome amidst the clamor of other voices. As one person said, "there are moments when I can lift above the fog. And this is one of those moments, talking to you. . . . it's just that feeling of someone taking all of their time to devote to you."

Several individuals entrusted us with secrets. One person wrote in a letter, "Linda, I don't know what to do next or who to turn to. . . . I'm very ashamed. . . . You are the only person I could think of to try to explain these problems, or to get some advice on what I should do. I have always more or less been a weak-minded, low-self-esteem person and very shy. . . . I've never mentioned it to the doctors or anybody." Others said, "Nobody knows about it but me and you," or, "I haven't told anyone else but you about this," in reference to symptoms. This sort of disclosure reinforced repeatedly our sense of the loneliness of these individuals, the lack of empathic others in their lives, our inabilities to fill this role, and increased puzzlement about how a person might respond if they saw their secrets on the printed page.

The opportunity to give voice to their complaints, fears, and hopes, and to account for themselves in their own terms was an important element in the research process. In some way, the interview can be seen as a positive end in and of itself. In another, it creates a responsibility to deliver the messages we receive. For example:

[interviewer notes] K. was concerned that I understand what he was telling me. He stated clearly that he does not talk freely about the spirits to other people because they don't understand. "I want you to understand. Everybody knows psychologists can take a channeler and tear them up bad." He seemed comfortable, perhaps even relieved to be able to talk about these things.

[interviewer notes] At the beginning of the interview H. remarked that the interview would help him too because he could talk. . . . H. was very talkative and willing to share more than the interview necessitated. He was very interested in the interview questions. He started off sitting across from me, and started reading the questions along with me. By the end of the interview, he was standing beside me, propping himself up on the table with his elbows and reading each question quietly after I read it. H. enjoyed the interview and agreed to follow-up interviews. He said he would even do them without pay. He commented that he enjoyed using his mind.

[interviewer notes] Although she was extremely anxious at first about the purpose of the interview, and why she had been chosen, she responded well to fairly extensive reassurances. Once the interview had begun, she was very talkative. . . . She has strong feelings about a number of incidents that have occurred while she was in various hospitals, and it was this that she was most particularly anxious to communicate about.

Another said simply, "It makes me feel better to know there are people who care about mental illness."

Summing Up

It has been my intention here to identify and describe some of the pleasures and perils of the work of chronic illness narratives. Some of the issues I have raised may be specific to work with individuals who have mental illnesses, but I believe many pertain to the larger population of individuals with enduring, disabling conditions.

When we engage in producing knowledge about persons with chronic illness, first and foremost we enter into a *relationship* with a person who may be vulnerable, impaired, pained, and lonely. Others with whom we work are courageous, defiant, triumphant, and functioning quite well. We create obligations and incur responsibilities when we enter into this process/relationship with these people. That the relationship is the fulcrum of this whole business was never more apparent than when in 1987 I began a ten-year follow-up of the people with whom I worked in 1975–77. The most difficult part of the uniformly warm and friendly reunions was the comparisons they made between themselves and me over the decade—how they measured their own stasis, loss, and (too rarely) gain over that time in relation to what had occurred in my life (a Ph.D., a book, tenure, money).

We also have responsibilities and obligations to those who fund our work, to our professions, and to the institutions and colleagues who give us access to those from whom we learn. Another essay would be required to discuss these concerns, and those that arise with regard to the relatives and significant others of our primary informants. Balancing and fulfilling all of these is as daunting a task as it is impossible.

I believe that it is possible, however, to reduce exploitation and trespass, to minimize violation of individual rights, ethical principles, and reasonable expectations, and to conduct the work in a way that increases the opportunity for mutual benefit and reduces the chances for harms and wrongs. I do not think it is possible to work in complete collaboration, in actual equality, or in total accord or consensus with our informants. Nor am I certain that these are unassailably good goals.

The first victim of coming to terms with this kind of work has to be pretense. The pretense that we do no harm, and the pretense that we do only harm; the pretense that we cannot do things differently and the pretense that we must do things completely differently.

So-called human subjects work is never completed. The real work *begins* after the consent form is signed. The ways that we choose to know about persons with chronic illness sometimes stretch the ethical principles endorsed by our professions and, more importantly, that we endorse as individual scholars. How far our responsibilities go and what they are, what authority we do and do not rightly claim, and how we give proper voice to what we know and what informants tell us are all topics that deserve careful discussion and debate. That discussion too is never completed, and only begins here.

In Conclusion

Recently, a seminar in performance ethnography embarked on a collaborative project with a woman who had multiple personality disorder. According to two colleagues who related this incident, and with whose permission I retell it, the author of the narrative on which the performance was based had the consent and active collaboration of this individual for the project. The seminar participants spent much of the semester adapting the narrative for performance, and even sent revisions in the script back and forth to the author and his subject for clarification and verification. The woman had had a horrible childhood, punctuated by sexual and psychological abuse, and an adulthood marked by anguish, psychiatric treatment, and considerable sexual misadventure. During a brief rehearsal before the second performance, she appeared at the theater, out of control with humiliation and rage. She screamed that she had no idea that the performance would be so sexual in nature, that she was betrayed and misrepresented, mortified at her portrayal. Furniture was thrown and individuals were threatened physically. The cast crouched, sobbing in fear and remorse. The security police removed her forcibly. That performance was canceled, but the next night went on as scheduled. The woman's therapist attended that evening and said that her patient was deeply humiliated by her own outburst, refused to leave her house, and was ashamed and depressed.

How could this tragedy have been avoided? Was it possible for this person to consent to a process whose product she could not imagine? After all the contributions of the students, faculty, and the narrator to the production of the script, whose story was it, anyway?

Acknowledgments

The research on which this paper is based was supported by grant number MH 40314 from the National Institute of Mental Health (1986–1993), and a Junior Faculty Development Award from the University of North Carolina (1987). There were two sets of collaborators in this project: the research team with whom I have worked for the past six years; and the informants with whom I have been engaged since 1975. Bill Lachicotte, Linda Illingworth, Julia Benoit, and particularly Bob Ruth and Anna Johnston have been especially helpful in both identifying and helping to address many of the topics discussed here. Their interview notes and observations, and their editorial commentary have contributed much richness to the analysis. The informants wish to remain anonymous, though I wish they did not feel compelled to do so. None of them has read this paper. Each consented to participate in a research process that would result in scholarly papers and publications. I owe a large debt to Joan Cassell, whose friendship and passionate response to this chapter have immeasurably improved it and my thinking, and to the members of this extraordinary gathering whose wisdom, experience, and ideas have influenced my voice. Dena Plemmons, Soyini Madison, Beverly Long, Larry Churchill, Nancy King, and Nancy Gottovi contributed comments, resources, and the all-important encouragement to the work.

NOTES

1. While the critical literary analysis of ethnography and the self-critical gaze of anthropologists as producers of texts proceeds apace, and undoubtedly accounts for some of the impetus for my choice of topic, we leave this discourse to the margins in this paper. The interested reader should consult Marcus and Fischer (1986), Conquergood (1991,

1992), Personal Narratives Group (1989), and Patai (1991) for examples of this perspective and an update on progress made and lost.

2. With acknowledged indebtedness and similarity of purpose to Geertz's (1988) chapter, Being Here: Whose Life Is It Anyway?

3. There are arguments currently in the courts about the limits of narrative (journalistic) license, and disputes over the boundaries and nature of biography and autobiography. The recent debate about Anne Sexton's biography and the conduct of her biographer (and psychotherapist) is a case in point. Personhood is sometimes public, and open for public reconstruction (or destruction, as in politics), sometimes private, off-limits for comment or literary interpretation.

4. For example, I do not "own" my own published words—few of us retain the copyright to our own texts. Indeed, I must get the permission of my publisher or the publishers of journals that contain my words to reproduce them for teaching purposes.

5. In his recent collection of autobiographical essays, Leonard Kriegel (1991) has conveyed the essence of this contest for identity and authority over self: "People struggle not only to define themselves but to avoid being defined by others. But to be a cripple is to learn that one can be defined from outside. . . . What we invariably discover is that our true selves, our own inner lives, have been auctioned off so that we can be palatable rather than real. . . . the only thing we can be certain of is that the world would prefer to turn a blind eye and a deaf ear to our real selves—and that it will do precisely that until we impose those selves on the world." The idea that there is a true, real, inner life/self that can be imposed on others turns symbolic interactionism on its ear—and epitomizes the self as a consciously contested entity.

6. Geertz (1988:131) classifies these somewhat differently as "deconstructive attacks on canonical works, and the very idea of canonicity as such; *Ideologiekritik* unmasking of anthropological writings as the continuation of imperialism by other means; clarion calls for reflexivity, dialogue, heteroglossia, linguistic play, linguistic self-consciousness, performative translation, verbatim recording, and first-person narrative as a form of cure."

REFERENCES

American Anthropological Association. 1971. Statements on Ethics: Principles of Professional Responsibility. (Amended October 1990.)

American Psychiatric Association. 1986. "Principles of Medical Ethics with Annotations Especially Applicable to Psychiatry." In Rena A. Gorlin, ed., *Codes of Professional Responsibility*. Washington, D.C.: Bureau of National Affairs. pp. 129–135.

American Psychological Association. 1989. Ethical Principles of Psychologists. Directory of the American Psychological Association. Vol. 1.

Barnard, David. 1985. "Unsung Questions of Medical Ethics." *Social Science and Medicine* 21(3): 243–249.

Barrett, Robert J. 1988. "Clinical Writing and the Documentary Construction of Schizophrenia." *Culture, Medicine, and Psychiatry* 12(3) 265–299.

Bouricius, Jean. 1989. "Negative Symptoms and Emotions in Schizophrenia." *Schizophrenia Bulletin* 15(2): 201–208.

Brody, Howard. 1987. *Stories of Sickness.* New Haven: Yale University Press.

Campbell, Jean. 1991. Toward Undiscovered Country. Ph.D. dissertation, University of California–Irvine.

Capron, A. M. 1991. "Protection of Research Subjects: Do Special Rules Apply in Epidemiology?" *Law, Medicine and Health Care* 19(3–4) Fall–Winter: 184–190.

Chamberlin, Judy. 1978. *On Our Own.* New York: McGraw Hill.

Charmaz, Kathy. 1987. "Struggling for a Self: Identity Levels of the Chronically Ill." *Research in the Sociology of Health Care* 6: 283–321.

———. 1983. "Loss of Self: a fundamental form of suffering in the chronically ill." *Sociology of Health and Illness* 5(2): 168–195.

Churchill, Larry. 1980. "Physician-Investigator/Patient-Subject: Exploring the Logic and the Tension." *The Journal of Medicine and Philosophy* 5(3): 215–224.

Churchill, Larry, and Sandra Churchill. 1982. "Storytelling in Medical Arenas: the art of self-determination." *Literature and Medicine* 1: 73–79.

Comaroff, Jean, and John Comaroff. 1991. *Of Revelation and Revolution.* Volume 1. Chicago: University of Chicago Press.

Conquergood, Dwight. 1992. "Ethnography, Rhetoric, and Performance." *Quarterly Journal of Speech* 78: 1–23.

———. 1991. Rethinking Ethnography: Towards a Critical Cultural Politics. Communication Monographs, Volume 58, June 1991.

Conrad, Peter. 1987. "The Experience of Illness: Recent and New Directions." *Research in the Sociology of Health Care* 6: 1–31.

Crapanzano, Vincent. 1980. *Tuhami: Portrait of a Moroccan.* Chicago: University of Chicago Press.

Davis, Dena. 1991. "Rich Cases: The Ethics of Thick Description." *The Hastings Center Report* 12–17. July–August.

Dickens, Bernard M., Larry Gostin, and Robert J. Levine. 1991. "Research on Human Populations: National and International Ethical Guidelines." *Law, Medicine and Health Care* 19(3–4) Fall–Winter: 157–161.

Dula, Annette. 1991. "Toward an African-American Perspective on Bio-Ethics." *Journal of Health Care for the Poor and Underserved* 2(2) Fall: 259–269.

Estroff, Sue E. 1985. *Making It Crazy: An Ethnography of Psychiatric Clients in an American Community.* Berkeley: University of California Press (paperback edition).

Estroff, Sue E., and John S. Strauss. 1989. "Epilogue: Forward." *Schizophrenia Bulletin* 15(2): 323.

Estroff, Sue E., et al. 1991. "Everbody's Got a Little Mental Illness: Accounts of Illness and Self Among Persons with Severe, Persistent Mental Illness." *Medical Anthropology Quarterly* 5(4): 331–369.

Fine, Michelle, and Adrienne Asch, eds. 1988. *Women with Disabilities: Essays in Psychology, Culture, and Politics*. Philadelphia: Temple University Press.

Frank, Gelya. 1988. "On Embodiment: A Case Study of Congenital Limb Deficiency in American Culture." In M. Fine and A. Asch, eds., *Women with Disabilities*. Philadelphia: Temple University Press. pp. 41–71.

———. 1979. "Finding the Common Denominator: A phenomenological critique of life history method." *Ethos* 7(1): 68–94.

Geertz, Clifford. 1988. *Works and Lives: The Anthropologist as Author*. Stanford, CA: Stanford University Press.

———. 1973. *The Interpretation of Cultures*. New York: Basic Books.

Gostin, Larry. 1991. "Ethical Principles for the Conduct of Human Subject Research: Population-Based Research and Ethics." *Law, Medicine and Health Care* 19(3–4) Fall–Winter: 191–201.

Jackson, Michael. 1989. *Paths Toward a Clearing: Radical Empiricism and Ethnographic Inquiry*. Bloomington: Indiana University Press.

Jeffries, J. J., E. Plummer, M. V. Seeman, and J. F. Thornton. 1990. *Living and Working with Schizophrenia*. Foreward and pp. 99–128. Toronto: University of Toronto Press.

Jennings, Bruce, Daniel Callahan, and Arthur L. Caplan. 1988. "Ethical Challenges of Chronic Illness." *Hastings Center Report* 1–16. February–March.

Johannsen, Agneta. 1992. "Applied Anthropology and Post-Modernist Ethnography." *Human Organization* 51(1): 71–81.

King, Nancy M. P., and Ann Folwell Stanford. 1992. "Patient Stories, Doctor Stories, and True Stories: A Cautionary Reading." *Literature and Medicine* 11: 185–199.

Kleinman, Arthur. 1988. *The Illness Narratives*. New York: Basic Books.

Kriegel, Leonard. 1991. *Falling Into Life*. Berkeley, CA: North Point Press.

Levine, Robert J. 1991. "Informed Consent: Some Challenges to the Universal Validity of the Western Model." *Law, Medicine and Health Care* 19(3–4) Fall–Winter: 207–213.

Lévi-Strauss, Claude. 1967. *Triste Tropiques*. John Russel, trans. New York: Antheneum.

Liebow, Elliot. 1993. *Tell Them Who I Am*. New York: The Free Press.

Marcus, George W., and Michael M. Fischer. 1986. *Anthropology as Cultural Critique: An Experimental Moment in the Human Sciences*. Chicago: University of Chicago Press.

Marshall, Patricia A. 1992. "Anthropology and Bioethics." *Medical Anthropology Quarterly* 6(1): 49–73.

McCarthy, Charles R., and Joan P. Porter. 1991. "Confidentiality: The Protection of Personal Data in Epidemiological and Clinical Research Trials." *Law, Medicine and Health Care* 19(3–4) Fall–Winter: 238–241.

McLean, Athena. 1990. "Contradictions in the Social Production of Clinical Knowledge: The Case of Schizophrenia." *Social Science and Medicine* 30(9): 969–985.

Murphy, Robert. 1989. *The Body Silent.* New York: Holt.

Patai, Daphne. 1991. "U.S. Academics and Third World Women: Is Ethical Research Possible?" In Sherna Berger Gluck and Daphne Patai, eds., *Women's Words: The Feminist Practice of Oral History.* New York: Routledge.

Personal Narratives Group, eds. 1989. *Interpreting Women's Lives.* Bloomington: Indiana University Press.

Peterson, Paul, ed. 1982. *A Mad People's History of Madness.* Pittsburgh: University of Pittsburgh Press.

Rabinow, Paul. 1977. *Reflections on Fieldwork in Morocco.* Berkeley: University of California Press.

Ratey, John J., Steven Sands, and Gillian Driscoll. 1986. "The Phenomenology of Recovery in a Chronic Schizophrenic." *Psychiatry* 49 (November): 277–289.

Reinharz, Shulamit. 1992. *Feminist Methods in Research.* New York: Oxford University Press.

Stoller, Robert J. 1988. "Patients' Responses to Their Own Case Reports." *Journal of the American Psychoanalytic Assn.* 36(2): 371–391.

Strauss, John. 1989. "Subjective Experiences of Schizophrenia." *Schizophrenia Bulletin* 15(2): 179–188.

Styron, William. 1990. *Darkness Visible.* New York: Random House.

Vonnegut, Mark. 1975. *The Eden Express.* New York: Basic Books.

Zola, Irving K. 1991. "Bringing Our Bodies and Ourselves Back In: Reflections on a Past, Present and Future Medical Sociology." *Journal of Health and Social Behavior* 32 (March): 1–16.

———. 1982. *Missing Pieces.* Philadelphia: Temple University Press.

PART TWO

6

BEYOND RESPECT TO RECOGNITION AND DUE REGARD

RONALD A. CARSON

There was a thing in us both that moved us in each other's direction, that
made us recognizable to each other. Whatever our complications, this
obdurate fact remained.[1]

The patient is always on the brink of revelation, and he needs someone
who can recognize it when it comes.[2]

As CONTEMPORARY BIOMEDICAL ethics has evolved conceptually, the principle of
respect for persons, and, in particular, respect for the autonomy of individual patients, has been given more weight than it can bear. This has come about as a consequence of the near unanimity among bioethicists in the view that medicine in
mass societies is a practice among moral strangers.[3] The argument is that because
patients and physicians in societies such are ours are moral strangers, a climate of
suspicion prevails. Not knowing what to expect of doctors, patients must assert
their right to self-determination. Only if they stipulate the terms of their contract
for care can they expect those terms to be met.

The principle of respect is unquestionably central to a sound medical ethic and
it must be steadily reinforced if it is to bear up under unrelenting economic and
technologic pressures that threaten to erode it. But in contemporary biomedical
ethics this principle does largely negative work. It reminds us to mind our own
business, to leave each other alone. That is sometimes necessary advice in medicine, especially in acute care medicine. But without a corresponding conception
of care that shows us how to be *with* each other in sickness as in health, some

requirement of responsiveness beyond calculation, the principle of respect is a prescription for abandonment of patients to a vacuous "freedom of choice."[4]

We have settled for too shallow an understanding of respect.[5] Certainly we should refrain from interfering in each others' lives when that is called for, but the ill are due regard as well as negative respect. They have attentiveness and considerateness coming as well as forbearance. Morally sound medical practice is not sustainable as "stranger medicine." Dialogue is required and, especially in dealing with chronic illness and disabling conditions, an acquired sense of familiarity with the patient's plight and life that eschews both clinical distance and frank familiarity.[6]

My aim here is to characterize that sense of familiarity by asking of some poems and stories of chronic sickness and disability what they can teach those who are not now, not yet, chronically ill or disabled about how to be with those who are. I will be thinking primarily of health care professionals, and my approach will be readerly rather than argumentative. Several books have been especially useful to me as I have thought about appropriate kinds of care for people with chronic illness and chronic disabling conditions. It is principally with some poets and with the authors of three books—Clara Claiborne Park, John Berger, and Arthur Frank—that I will be conversing in what follows. Some of these sources reveal another's experience in the first person, others describe moments of recognition on the part of a third person—an observer, a narrator. In each instance, the sources are texts, which is to say representations of experience. The first-person accounts, too, are crafted disclosures, not interior monologues, and we, the interpreters, whether at one remove or more, are invited to "read" the characters presented as "images of possible people."[7] Each of my interlocutors reveals a clue that can guide us beyond negative respect to regard for people with chronic illnesses and disabilities. The clue's name is "recognition."

Stories and poetry persuade by telling and evoking rather than by exhorting or arguing. To tell is to rehearse, and to recount and reveal. To tell a tale is to disclose experience so that its significance is discernible. Poems and stories are often not transparent to meaning; to make sense of them requires a studied attentiveness alternating with an openness to possibility. Evidence is sorted and weighed. The past is probed, the present described, the future imagined. In this process insights take form in the imagination. As a plausible reading of a poem or a story begins to dawn, the interpreter asks of the text Is this what it's like, how it feels to be in this character's shoes?—and pays careful attention, keeping the case open all the while.[8] It is the same with doctors and patients. This pair of poems by James Dickey suggests how this is so.

Angina

That one who is the dreamer lies mostly in her left arm,
Where the pain shows first,
Tuned in on the inmost heart,
Never escaping. On the blue, bodied mound of chenille,
That limb lies still.
Death in the heart must be calm,

Must not look suddenly, but catch the windowframed squirrel
In a mild blue corner
Of an eye staring straight at the ceiling
And hold him there.
Cornered also, the oak tree moves
All the ruffled green way toward itself

Around the squirrel thinking of the sun
As small boys and girls tiptoe in
Overawed by their existence,
For courtly doctors long dead
Have told her that to bear children
Was to die, and they are the healthy issue

Of four of those. Oh, beside that room the oak leaves
Burn out their green in an instant, renew it all
From the roots when the wind stops.
All afternoon she dreams of letters
To disc jockeys, requesting the "old songs,"
The songs of the nineties, when she married and caught

With her first child rheumatic fever.
Existence is family: sometime,
Inadequate ghosts round the bed,
But mostly voices, low voices of serious drunkards
Coming in with the night light on
And the pink radio turned down;

She hears them ruin themselves
On the rain-weeping wires, the bearing-everything poles,
Then dozes, not knowing sleeping from dying—
It is day. Limbs stiffen when the heart beats
Wrongly. Her left arm tingles,
The squirrel's eye blazes up, the telephone rings,

Her children and her children's children fail
In school, marriage, abstinence, business.

But when I think of love
With the best of myself—that odd power—
I think of riding, by chairlift,
Up a staircase burning with dust

In the afternoon sun slanted also
Like stairs without steps
To a room where an old woman lies
Who can stand on her own two feet
Only six strange hours every month:
Where such a still one lies smiling

And takes her appalling risks
In absolute calm, helped only by the most
Helplessly bad music in the world, where death,
A chastened, respectful presence
Forced by years of excessive quiet
To be stiller than wallpaper roses,

Waits, twined in the roses, saying slowly
To itself, as sprier and sprier
Generations of disc jockeys chatter,
I must be still and not worry,
Not worry, not worry, to hold
My peace, my poor place, my own.[9]

Angina, a throttling spasm, a painful sense of suffocation in the chest, secondary in this case to rheumatic fever in early adulthood. Now three additional children and some grandchildren later, having outlived the doctors who warned her of the life-and-death risk of bearing more children, this brave woman lies calmly beneath the tufted spread in her upstairs bedroom, attuned to the palaver of deejays and to the beating of her damaged heart.

She knows from years of experience that death is never more than a heartbeat away and that when its approach is signaled by pain in the left arm, calm and concentration are called for. She must avoid sudden movements, fix her gaze on the ceiling, and hold still at the periphery of her vision the bushy-tailed animal in the oak tree just outside the window whose life is all jerk and jump. Hold still, too, the tree itself whose branches waft in the wind—until the pain passes, and the leaves, having burnt themselves out in an instant, are renewed from the roots. Only then can she return to her reveries and to auditing the ups and downs of her family's life until the advent of the next erratic heartbeat, the tingling in the arm, the squirrel's eye wide, signaling danger.

As the title announces, this is a poem about chronic, erratic pain and the threat of death. But when the poet thinks of love he thinks of rising to another level, literally "riding, by chairlift, Up a staircase burning with dust In the afternoon sun slanted also Like stairs without steps" but also figuratively, ascending a smooth sun shaft to a room where the ailing dreamer can rise from her bed only very occasionally but who has risen above her condition to a kind of contentment. Cornered by her condition, she takes her risks calmly, one day at a time, thereby keeping death in its place. Death is woven into the tapestry of her life, ever near but mostly unnoticeable. Death, too, has been forced to learn patience. When the poet thinks of love he thinks of this disabled dreamer enduring and smiling.

Buckdancer's Choice

So I would hear out those lungs,
The air split into nine levels,
Some gift of tongues of the whistler

In the invalid's bed: my mother,
Warbling all day to herself
The thousand variations of one song;

It is called Buckdancer's Choice.
For years, they have all been dying
Out, the classic buck-and-wing men

Of traveling minstrel shows;
With them also an old woman
Was dying of breathless angina,

Yet still found breath enough
To whistle up in my head
A sight like a one-man band,

Freed black, with cymbals at heel,
An ex-slave who thrivingly danced
To the ring of his own clashing light

Through the thousand variations to one song
All day to my mother's prone music,
The invalid's warbler's note,

While I crept close to the wall
Sock-footed, to hear the sounds alter,
Her tongue like a mockingbird's break

Through stratum after stratum of a tone
Proclaiming what choices there are
For the last dancers of their kind,

For ill women and for all slaves
Of death, and children enchanted at walls
With brass-beating glow underfoot,

Not dancing but nearly risen
Through barnlike, theaterlike houses
On the wings of the buck and wing.[10]

Here two images of performance are joined. We are brought to the bedside of the poet's invalid mother whistling countless variations of a song called Buck-dancer's Choice. Buckdancers were minstrels of the American South who danced a jig by tapping out a clattering rhythm on a stage. "For years," we are told, "they have all been dying Out, the classic buck-and-wing men"—recognizably buck-and-wing men by their two-toned black and white wingtipped cordovans to which tiny brass cymbals were attached at the heel.

Breathless with angina, the woman's self-absorbed whistling conjures up in her son's imagination such a man, once enslaved, now free to dance and choose. His mother too, though bound to bed, finds "breath enough" to whistle, to warble as songbirds do, trilling away, improvising and mocking her own condition by choosing a "thousand variations of one song." Never mind that there is only one song, one bedfast life, still there are choices. That is what she celebrates—her choice, Buckdancer's Choice. And her defiant music-making so enchants her sock-footed son that he begins to see how she survives. "Not dancing but nearly risen" on the wings of song.

In these poems, living with a chronic life-threatening condition means not recovery but perseverance, personal renewal, and a kind of serene defiance. Is something similar possible in other circumstances where the body has been irremediably damaged? Let's look at a trilogy of poems about stroke.

Stroke

Eyes into which life after life
had disappeared: faces of children, of women
not always easy to walk away from
or toward. Propped on hospital pillows
he spoke right through you

to people not there,
pored over strange lines
in his hands, wandered the shore and inlets
of odd tea-colored stains on the ceiling
while our whole family took turns
watching his thought slowly close
like an infant's skull,
or gates of a town whose exiles
are never forgiven.

And is each face he looks into
three-quarters memory?
Like dawn's pink problem,
an echo? If our own everyday sky-color
has an endless bend in it
which night straightens out
then returns, his head toward the window
stares through ninety years of spring rains
the catalpa roots and oak limbs
have diagrammed, hears family names arriving
quietly, from further away than ever,
hears "Rachel" as word: no longer a wish,
no longer the bride still half girl
opening both arms, like summer roads
that loved being taken.

Twice daily you chattered,
nothing we knew could distract him.
Instead he looked at his hands
as if weighing what used to be theirs
and how long they had held it.[11]

The dominant mood here is one of sadness over loss. A man is there in the presence of his family but has lost his way. His eyes look but are vacant. He studies the map of his palms, the lifelines leading nowhere. He tries to read the tea leaves but divines no direction. It is as if the faces of those who appear before him disappear into his eyes as into an emptiness. You feel hollow as he speaks through you to an absence, perhaps someone he mistakes you for. Is he hallucinating? Or remembering? His wife's name when uttered registers as a word only, detached from desire. His life no longer comes full circle like ours with a dawn followed by day and the return of night. Instead it is just here, inexplicably, a linear, trackless now. As his family keeps its sad vigil they talk to him, but he seems permanently preoccupied, locked into his life, trying to recollect he knows not what.

Anna's Grace

And with damp rags she bathes him,
brings him his whiskey in the evenings,
says the rosary before the crucifix
and dried palm leaves on the wall.
He can't stand by himself
or walk or lift his arms.
He doesn't know the children
or grandchildren who come to his bed
to hold his swollen hands
and kiss his face. On the plain
of stroke he sleeps in the day bed
where the sun may find him
and the toilet isn't far
when she must carry him
in to piss because he can't
hold his cock, so she holds it
for him, as when in love
they'd tumbled into the same bed.
He lies in the consuming
shock of the brain assaulting
itself and calls in the language
he would not abandon
to the country
dying out in his heart.
And the old woman
who shaves him
with such grace he doesn't bleed,
sleeps on the hard couch,
flashlight on the table beside her
so she may shine and move
the light under her blankets
when he demands at night to see
no other man sleeps with her.[12]

Here is a man stranded on the level, landmarkless "plain of stroke." He does not know his offspring. He speaks in a diminished vocabulary of demand and complaint. He lives by the grace of Anna, his long-suffering companion, who bathes him, brings him drink, says devotions, carries him to the bathroom, allays the suspicion that has displaced desire, and "shaves him with such grace he doesn't bleed. . . . " Anna's "grace" is her carefulness, her devotion, her unrequitable gift.

Someone Else

When she had come to live with them, by then
vanity was all her stroke had left her.
Yet it became another kind of health,
a way to get through days when she would wake
in her wet bed, a child again, afraid
she might be found before the sheets were clean;
or showering, when she would have to see her body
like someone else resisting her, so stiff
it only let her turn enough to reach,
not wash, the bitter smell that clung like shame.

So she would spend the mornings struggling
with her silk slip and dress, and work her stockings
up her legs till they seemed agile with shimmering.
The rouged cheek, the hair done up, the nails
polished till the brightness made her hands
(if only they'd keep still) less like a stranger's—
these enabled her to leave her room
and face them, and believe the care she needed
was what they owed her,
what she permitted them to give. They were,

she would tell herself, tottering her great
weight down the stairs, no better than her husbands,
those first betrayers: the sullen courtesy
her grandchild showed, the irritation hiding
in her daughter's pity, she could at least ignore them
(at least there would be power there), and wait
till they went out, wanting them out,
so she could feel finally at home,
the tv on,
just her and her celebrities.

She could anticipate each set response,
each misery. Nothing could surprise her.
And with a kind of joy she could be certain
that even if some star walked from the screen

the mirror, always at hand, would show her hair
in place, her face powdered; she could feel
the aftertaste of mouthwash, could even savor
the bitter cleanness of her mouth, and know,
nearly invincible, that she was ready,
should anybody come to take her out.[13]

She is a mother and grandmother who, betrayed by her body, has come to live
with her daughter's family. It is an arrangement dictated by necessity. She needs
their care but resents it. They pity her and tolerate her, all the while wishing it
weren't so. She maintains a kind of control over a life unexpectedly thrust upon
her by putting necessity to work for her, in *allowing* her family to provide the care
she needs. In a body grown strange and resistant, it is vanity that lets her come
out at all and settle down to watch the reassuringly predictable soaps. Her vanity
is "another kind of health" that gets her through days of shame and bitterness.
More than this there is "a kind of joy" in the certainty that if a celebrity were to
step from the screen (or if death were to announce itself?) she would be composed, well-groomed, ready to go out.

There is no enchantment here. Pacing oneself is not an option; the heart is not
the injured part here. It is the mind and voluntary motion that are compromised.
There is defiance, grace, reconciliation, and a sad watchfulness.

Watchfulness blurs into wistfulness when the poet, contemplating a mentally
disturbed child, yearns for the tide to turn but knows it will not.

Jenny

You see it's that she can't remember songs
and when friends come to play and want to sing,
you know, songs that children always sing,
she can't remember the songs she sang
even the day before, songs all children sing.

She plays with younger ones,
one little girl really,
and she is so much quicker than my child
and screams at her and calls her stupid
because she can't remember songs.

She can ice skate,
and there's nothing wrong with her balance,

and so she glides and looks sad and bewildered
at those who can both skate and sing,
songs that all children know and sing.

And when she is older and the songs are harder
and she needs songs to sing
if she is hurt or loves or isn't sure,
what will she do;
my child who can't remember songs.[14]

Cut off from song—songs of consolation, songs of celebration and doubt—how could we say how it hurts, or that we love, or that we're not sure? Everyone knows how to sing such songs, everyone but Jenny. The poet's helplessness in the face of his child's inability to remember songs is despairing.

Waiting

The best place, when he is fractious,
is the British Museum, Egyptian Room.

There she sits on a bench
waiting for him, waiting for the time to pass.

She has waited for him in surgeries,
in special schools, in workshops;

waited for signs of improvement;
for the tide to turn.

Now he is peering at the embalmed animals
close-bandaged in their leak-marked linen.

He knocks on the glass with his knuckle
at the skinny cat sitting up tall,

the baby bull, the ducks and,
next to the crocodile, his own face

matching grin for grin. He raps harder
and she takes his arm.

Leave them alone. They won't wake up.
Hand in hand they walk away down the stairs,

out past the pillars. She winds his scarf
tightly round him against the cold.[15]

We are brought to the Egyptian Room of the British Museum. The full significance of this choice of place will be shortly disclosed by the poet (poets do not make such selections at random; neither do patients). There "she" waits for "him"—apparently a mother waiting for her son, though, significantly, the relationship is never described and the two people who populate the poem are never identified. She also waits for time to pass. The impression created is that the time for hope is past. The clinic visits, the attempts at rehabilitation have been exhausted. Through those she waited, hoping. Now she bides her time and thinks of ways to occupy him when he is unruly, like visiting the Egyptian Room. There he looks searchingly at the mummified animals, well-preserved but lifeless, bearing signs of the life that has seeped from their bodies. When he mirrors the crocodile's idiot grin and bangs on the glass to wake the dull menagerie, she loses patience, explaining, "They won't wake up," and takes him by the arm out of the Egyptian Room. As they exit the museum her irritation seems to have subsided. They are holding hands. As they step into the outside air she (his "Mummy") moves in motherly fashion to protect him from the cold. All that remains is to brace against the cold. As "She winds his scarf tightly around him . . . " we realize that for her he is as though embalmed.

Mary, too, is retarded but destined for affection and wholeness.

Mary

Mary's body blossomed, out of step
with her forever-a-child's brain.

Sometimes a perfect stillness
heralded an ungainly jig,

teeth sunk in her wrist to offer
the glistening foundations of a ring of ancient stones.

Her brother and I took her to school
through jokes and catcalls and worse:

the day when an insensitive teacher,
asking who we would marry, included Mary.

I want our David, she said.
I bit my lip as the question returned:

Why Mary of course.
Their laughter was sharper, my blood sweet.

At twelve she was sent to a Home.
Her brother went to visit and said there was a dance

where her partner was a gangling boy
with lost, up-staring eyes.

She helped him through a clumsy, shuffling waltz
but there was no one there to laugh,

they were turning in a place where all are mended,
on that mist-clearing solstice morning

when flower-crowned figures move
to a gentle, measured beat.[16]

The movement of this poem is from awkwardness to gracefulness, from being ungainly and out of step to stepping to a "gentle, measured beat." Mary's behavior has a primitive cast and is inscrutable (the "ring of ancient stones" revealed when she bites her wrist to the bone). But she makes good sense to her father when in class she singles out her brother as the person she would most like to marry. When her father bites his lip in anxious anticipation of his daughter's response, the blood is sweet. Her classmates laugh, her teacher is patronizing, but her father recognizes the logic of the choice of a companion who has taken her to school "through jokes and catcalls and worse. . . . " Sometime later, following a visit to the Home where Mary now lives, her brother reports on a dance where she helped her partner drag his slow feet through a waltz and no one laughed—because Mary and her partner were moving in a gentle gyre around a point of perfect stillness, a movement not ungainly but measured. All bewilderment was lifting away. "They were turning in a place where all are mended." Healing is more than remedy. Mary's brain is "forever-a-child's" but as she dances her life is mended.

Even when mending is out of reach, reconciliation may not be, as in these two poems about arthritic pain.

The Knitted Glove

You come into my office wearing a blue
knitted glove with a ribbon at the wrist.
You remove the glove slowly, painfully,
and dump out the contents, a worthless hand.
What a specimen! It looks much like a regular hand,
warm, pliable, soft, you can move the fingers.

If it's not one thing, it's another.
Last month the fire in your hips had you down
or up mincing across the room with a cane.
When I ask about the hips today, you pass it off
so I can't tell if only the pain
or the memory is gone. The knitted hand
is the long and short of it, pain doesn't exist
in the past any more than this morning does.

This thing, the name for your solitary days,
for the hips, the hand, for the walk of your eyes
away from mine, this thing is coyote, a trickster.
I want to call, "Come out, you son of a dog!"
and wrestle that name to the ground for you,
I want to take its neck between my hands.
But in this world I don't know how to find
the bastard, so we sit. We talk about the pain.[17]

The contents of the knitted glove look, feel, and move like a regular hand, but when dumped out for the doctor to examine, this hand is seen to be without value, a mere specimen of pain. The pain is crafty, carnivorous, stealing from hip to hand, feeding on flesh and lying low. (Worthless goods are "dumped"; coyotes scour trash dumps for scraps.) The doctor wants to subdue the pain, exorcise the intruder by naming it, but he cannot find it (" . . . you son of a dog"—literally, a coyote, but also, as expletive, "you son-of-a-bitch"). He wants to take the beast in his healthy hands and strangle it for the patient's sake, but it is not "there" like that. So he listens to the patient talk about the pain.

The poet, too, listens to the barmaid as she tells him what it's like and how she lives with bones outlined by pain.

A Few Carats of Pain

The shadows were roaring
With pain on the other side of the mirror,
She pushed the glass up against the optic
But called the barman to draw my beer;
'You lose your grip', she said,
'In rheumatoid arthritis, which is
Stone in the garden of the joints',
She explained, and in the east wind

As if ice in the air were condensing on this stone,
Black ice; 'Verglas?' She agreed.

Welding in the glass,
Immovable joints under construction
On the other side of the mirror,
Shadows arced out on the face.
She served me chaser whisky anodyne
And the barman drew my beer in his firm grip.
'That's a handsome stone, my dear . . . '
'It's my life-savings, lover-boy,
Small as it is . . . ' among the calcite flowers
Like an arc-tooth in the garden, refracting pain;
'You lose your grip at first
And no sign can be seen except the pain,
So I bought the diamond
To wear on my arthritic hand.' It was like
A folded window into the skin,
It was like a point of pain
Held on a gold band of concentration,
Its interior shadowless.

Her hand, she says, is a garden to this star
Which is a precipice when the east wind blows
And you lose your grip; you know your bones
In this disease, she says, outlined with pain,
'I've crowned this one like a King
With my life-savings . . . '; she pushed
My glass up into the whisky-spring, and smiled;
Her perfume filled the bar, her story gripped us.[18]

Though hampered, hers is no worthless hand. She can push a glass up against the upturned whisky bottle. Even this costs her though, as the customer can clearly see in the grimace reflected in the mirror opposite both of them behind the optic. She calls the barman to draw his beer, explains that rheumatoid arthritis prevents her from gripping the tap handle, and searches for a likeness—stone in the garden of the joints, ice, black ice condensing on the stone. Trying to comprehend, the customer ventures an analogy of his own: "Verglas?" Is it like a glazing of the joints, like fusing them? Yes, like that.

She explains further that although rheumatoid arthritis is invisible, "You lose your grip" on things like the tap handle, on life. To symbolize the pain, to make it visible, she has invested her life savings in a small diamond ring which crowns her arthritic hand—a regal, life-saving device, she explains, as she serves the poet another shot and smiles.

Two final poems, these about recalcitrant bodies.

broken

> i don't cry because it was my favorite glass
> but squat here on the floor, tears forming
> because it is all so hard
> these days.
> to arrange
> my body down here
> this low. to lift
> the splinters and the arcs
> in dustpan, to transport them
> to a safer place.
> unexpected major chore
> in the scheme of a day.
> most of all i cry
> for the ice cubes
> dusty, melting on the floor
> for i craved cold water
> and they were all i had.[19]

Craving a glass of cold water, she goes to the freezer for ice cubes only to drop both, shattering them on the floor. Tears come not because the glass was her favorite, but "because it is all so hard these days." Getting her body down to floor level, assembling the splintered glass in a dustpan, carrying the dustpan to the trash can—a seemingly routine clean-up but an "unexpected major chore in the scheme of a day" for one whose body won't obey. Most of all the tears come at the sight of her only ice cubes melting on the floor. They were the only ones she had to quench her thirst. Her broken body too, is the only one she has. It, too, is "melting."

Song for My Son

> a wooden puppet with tangled
> strings   he bobs and bounces
> in mid-air   head flopping
> arms waving   my hands

under his arms sustain
his spastic stiffness
the Blue Fairy cradling
sweet Pinocchio
He loves to rock and roll
feet prancing   a crazy
puppet dance   his face glows
with the light   of the wishing
star   and borrowing his
brilliance   we too dance
heads bobbing   arms waving
faster and faster until
cast off puppets all
we fall to the floor   laughing
while the fading light
of the wishing star
caresses his face[20]

A fey, a fairy godmother, she steadies her son—sustains and cradles him—through a fitful rock and roll dance routine. His limbs wooden, his "strings" tangled, he dances up a storm, becomes luminous and is transported to a world where wishes come true. So joyous are his movements, so hilarious, so contagious, that they join in the puppet dance, "borrowing his brilliance," until they all collapse exhausted and laughing on the floor. And, though the light of the wishing star is fading, it caresses sweet Pinocchio's face as it dims.

In each of these poems there is a moment of recognition by virtue of which a life permanently damaged by disease or constrained by persistent pain is perceived to be liveable, if, at times of deepest despair, just barely so. Or the moment of recognition calls for watchfulness on the part of companions and caregivers. Such recognition is part insight, part acknowledgment—some appreciation of what it must be like to measure one's life by the erratic beat of one's heart, to care for a family member who has suffered a stroke, or to accommodate one's life to an unpredictable body—one's own or one's child's—and beyond this, a frank appreciation of the demands of such a life.

Clara Claiborne Park recalls a revelation that dawned on her when, after a bad experience with stateside psychiatrists, she sought help for her autistic daughter at Anna Freud's Hampstead Clinic and was received there with "healing kindness." It came to her then that

Before one feels great pain one may think—I thought—that one would want people not to notice, to aid one in the attempt to carry on—business here as usual. It is not so. Business may seem as usual but it is not. What one wants is that people should know that. What one wants is sympathy, understanding, not tacit but openly given. What one wants is love.[21]

Park characterizes earlier encounters with professionals as having gone awry, not because the professionals were not knowledgeable but because they lacked imagination. For almost four years, Park and her husband had been doing their best to bring up their hermetically isolated third child. Then they sought the help of specialists.

We expected to talk with wise and sympathetic people—wise because of a wide experience with sick children, sympathetic because it was their vocation to help those in trouble. We too had experience with a sick child, intense and prolonged if not wide, and we had been trying with every resource we possessed to help those in trouble—our baby, our normal children, ourselves. We were amateurs. They were professionals. But we had, we thought, a common task. Unconsciously we expected to be welcomed, not as patients, but as collaborators in the work of restoring this small, flawed spirit. We were doing something terribly hard, and we had been doing it quite alone. . . . We wanted information and techniques. We wanted sympathy—not the soppy kind; we were grown-up adults—but some evidence of fellow feeling . . . we wanted a little reassurance, a little recognition, a little praise.[22]

Of her English analyst Park says, "as no one else, she seemed to realize how hard my job was."[23]

This desire for recognition is echoed in Arthur Frank's account of his own double bout with illness. In the first round—a heart attack at 39—he and his doctor did not consider the personal import of what it was like to sense one's heart beating erratically and uncontrollably fast and then to fall down on the jogging path and pass out. Concentrating on the medical facts of the case, they unwittingly left the human significance of the experience out of the picture. Frank kept asking himself, "What's happening to me?" The cardiological details did not suffice, but neither did he know what else to ask. "*I did not know what I wanted to say* or what I wanted the physician to say. . . . I'm not sure that what I wanted to say could be put into words. But I needed some recognition of what was happening to me."[24] A year later, seeking out a third opinion on painful symptoms that corresponded to none of the results of routine tests, Frank learns from a specialist he has not met before that he may have testicular cancer.

> By then I felt less terrorized by the idea of cancer than validated by a recognition that I was seriously ill. . . . Even though my worst fears were realized in what he said, the physician showed, just by the way he looked at me and a couple of phrases he used, that he shared in the seriousness of my situation. The vitality of his support was as personal as it was professional.[25]

Emboldened by these signs of recognition, Frank could get down to the business of dealing with his illness and, as important if he was to survive whole, he could keep sight of himself in his illness. If the recognition he needed at the point of diagnosis was an acknowledgment of the seriousness of his situation, recognition's form would change as treatment began. Although in becoming a patient he had to learn dependence, he also worked at his role as lead actor in the drama of his illness. It was that for which he now desired recognition. This required a role reversal of considerable dimensions in a theater dominated by doctors, but it was necessary if Frank was ever to relinquish the role of patient and go into remission.

The drama metaphor is employed to good effect by John Berger in his sympathetic portrayal of Dr. John Sassal, making the rounds of his country parish. In his early years, after a stint as a Navy surgeon, Sassal played the part of lifesaver to his senior partner's role as curer of souls.

> He imagined himself as a sort of mobile one-man hospital. He performed appendix and hernia operations on kitchen tables. He delivered babies in caravans. It would almost be true to say that he sought out accidents. . . . He dealt only with crises in which he was the central character; or, to put it another way, in which the patient was *simplified* by the degree of his physical dependence on the doctor.[26]

Dr. Sassal matures and mellows as he becomes attuned to the rhythms of his adopted community. Over time he relinquishes his leading role to his patients and takes satisfaction in supporting roles as various as the dramas of all the lives of which he has become a part. To switch metaphors, he becomes "an honorary member of the family," a brother, to be precise. Berger explains:

> When I speak of a fraternal relationship—or rather of the patient's deep, unformulated expectation of fraternity—I do not of course mean that the doctor can or should behave like an actual brother. What is required of him is that he should recognize his patient with the certainty of an ideal brother. The function of fraternity is recognition.[27]

Illness exacerbates one's sense of difference to the point of loneliness. The task of the doctor is to recognize the patient. This task is carried out not only verbally, though words do matter, but also by the doctor's way of being with the patient.

(Recall Arthur Frank's reference to "the way he looked at me and a couple of phrases he used.") This requires an act of imagination.

> The patient must be given the chance to recognize, despite his aggravated self-consciousness, aspects of himself in the doctor, but in such a way that the doctor seems to be Everyman. This chance is probably seldom the result of a single exchange, and it may come about more as the result of the general atmosphere than of any special words said. As the confidence of the patient increases, the process of recognition becomes more subtle. At a later stage of treatment, it is the doctor's acceptance of what the patient tells him and the accuracy of his appreciation as he suggests how different parts of his life may fit together, it is this which then persuades the patient that he and the doctor and other men are comparable because whatever he says of himself or his fears or his fantasies seems to be at least as familiar to the doctor as to him. He is no longer an exception. He can be recognized. And this is the prerequisite for cure or adaptation.[28]

To break the circle of uniqueness closed by illness and to counter the sick person's magnified sense of his own dissimilarity, the doctor must present himself to patients as "a comparable man," admitting his likeness to them and his solidarity with them. There must be about him "the constant will of a man trying to recognize."[29] Only so may the patient become no longer an exception.

This turn of phrase is reminiscent of something Sallie Tisdale remarks in her portrait of life in a nursing home she calls Harvest Moon. Tisdale observes how the nurses and the aides there care for strangers from the streets "who have become no longer strangers."[30] No longer an exception, no longer strangers. "This," Tisdale notes, "it one of the meanings of community: recognition . . . [to] belong to a tribe of people both needing and giving, dependent and independent in turn."[31] Because our very identity as moral beings is shaped in significant measure by the reflection of ourselves mirrored back to us by others, recognition is not optional but is a necessary acknowledgment of our membership in a moral community.[32]

The subtext of this essay is that, though necessary, indeed nonnegotiable in relations between health care professionals and those who need their attention, respect, conceived negatively, is not enough. Regard is required as well, not as supererogation, but as a constitutive element of ordinary care, close to the heart of healing. It may seem odd to speak of healing in relation to chronic illness or disability, for surely healing implies recovery and chronic means lasting or recurring. Remissions notwithstanding, one does not get over chronic illness. And although one may be temporarily incapacitated by injury or disease, the term disability is usually reserved for permanent impairments. Nonetheless, upon reflection, these first impressions reveal themselves as half-truths, because healing is more than remedy.

This lesson is being relearned as the prevailing medical mentality slowly shifts away from so exclusive a concentration on rescue of the critically ill toward care for the chronically ill—from "flexed-muscle medicine,"[33] requiring a "doctor of stark emergency," to chronic care requiring professionals who possess a willingness to take part in a drama featuring the patient, and who have "an appetite for experience"[34] and an imagination capable of recognition, of appreciating others as they are. Will this shift in sensibility make for better ethical decision-making? Probably, but indirectly. It will do so by broadening the context of moral reflection to include not only respect, which aims to protect people from violation, but also regard, whose aim is recognition, affirmation, confirmation.

Acknowledgments

Every effort has been made to trace copyright for the poems included in this essay. The author gratefully acknowledges the following poems.

John Mann Astrachan. "Jenny" first appeared in "Letters to the Editor: Jenny" in *The New England Journal of Medicine*, May 27, 1982. Reprinted by permission.

Connie Bensley. "Waiting" is reprinted from *Central Reservations: New and Selected Poems* (Newcastle upon Tyne: Bloodaxe Books, 1990) and first appeared in the *Times Literary Supplement*, September 11–17, 1987. Reprinted by permission of the poet.

Jack Coulehan. "The Knitted Glove" first appeared in *On Doctoring*, Richard Reynolds and John Stone, eds. (New York: Simon and Schuster, 1991). Reprinted by permission of the poet.

Marilyn Davis. "Song for My Son" is reprinted from *Toward Solomon's Mountain: The Experience of Disability in Poetry*, Joseph L. Baird and Deborah S. Workman, eds. (Philadelphia, PA: Temple University Press, 1986). Reprinted by permission of the poet.

James Dickey. "Angina" and "Buckdancer's Choice" from *Buckdancer's Choice*, copyright 1965 by James Dickey. Published by Wesleyan University Press. Reprinted by permission of the University Press of New England.

Peter Redgrove. "A Few Carats of Pain" is reprinted from the *Times Literary Supplement*, March 20, 1987. Reprinted by permission.

Reg Saner. "Stroke" first appeared in *The Georgia Review*, Spring 1984. Reprinted by permission of the poet.

Alan Shapiro. "Someone Else" is reprinted from *The American Scholar*, Summer 1983.

David Sweetman. "Mary" is reprinted from the *Times Literary Supplement*, December 18–24, 1987.

Bruce Weigl. "Anna's Grace" first appeared in *The American Poetry Review*, 1990. Reprinted by permission of the poet.

zana. "broken" first appeared in *Toward Solomon's Mountain: The Experience of Disability in Poetry*, Joseph L. Baird and Deborah S. Workman, eds. (Philadelphia, PA: Temple University Press, 1986). Reprinted by permission of the poet.

NOTES

1. Richard Bausch, "Spirits," in *Spirits and Other Stories* (New York: Simon and Schuster, 1987), 237.

2. Anatole Broyard, "Doctor, Talk to Me," *The New York Times Magazine*, August 26, 1990, 36.

3. See James F. Childress and Mark Siegler, "Metaphors and Models of Doctor-Patient Relationships: Their Implications for Autonomy," *Theoretical Medicine* 5 (1984), 17–30; H. Tristram Engelhardt, Jr., "Bioethics in Pluralist Societies," *Perspectives in Biology and Medicine* 26 (Autumn 1982), 65–78; and Robert M. Veatch, "The Physician as Stranger: The Ethics of the Anonymous Patient-Physician Relationship," in Earl E. Shelp, ed., *The Clinical Encounter* (Dordrecht, Holland: D. Reidel, 1983), 187–207.

4. Robert A. Burt illuminates a dynamic of responsiveness in doctor-patient relations and shows how "the fallacy, the ultimate pretension, of the conception of the individual as socially isolated and rationally self-controlling" precipitates a disruption in the relationship that leaves the patient "wholly choice-making" and "utterly alone." *Taking Care of Strangers* (New York: The Free Press, 1979), 172, 118, 117.

5. See Daniel Callahan, "Minimalist Ethics," *The Hastings Center Report*, October 1981, 19–25; William F. May has observed that "ethicists do not adequately respect or protect the moral being of patients if they simply clear out a zone of indeterminate liberty free from medical interference but fail to lead the patient to discuss the moral uses to which the patient puts his liberty. . . . Respect must include a willingness to engage the patient

and the patient's family in a moral give and take, a sometimes painful mutual deliberation, judgment, and criticism, and an occasional accounting for one another's views, on both sides, in the professional exchange." *The Patient's Ordeal* (Bloomington: Indiana University Press, 1991), 207, note 2.

6. "Clinical distance" is the professional's (largely self-protective) posture in the presence of the patient as moral stranger. By "frank familiarity" I mean to distinguish behavior inappropriate to a professional relationship (such as pretending to be the patient's friend) from "a sense of familiarity," that is, a context for the patient's experience.

7. James Phelan, *Reading People, Reading Plots* (Chicago: University of Chicago Press, 1989), 2.

8. John Burt observes, "What moves us to assent to the fiction that characters are subjects as well as objects is perhaps not very different from what moves us to see other people as subjects, for after all somebody else's subjectivity is no more accessible to us than is the subjectivity of a fictional character. We take people in themselves only when we realize that what we know about them already does not answer or make irrelevant every other question we might ask about them. It is only the person whose reality it has not occurred to us to grant that we claim to fully understand, because only about such people can we claim to know all that we want to know. Only such people would we reduce to a formula or to that aspect in which we see them.

"Only when we prevent ourselves from saying that we understand someone do we stand back and accord that person the respect we wish to be given ourselves. We restrain our understanding, suspending not our judgment (for that goes on continuously) but rather our disposition to regard the case of that person as closed." John Burt, "Romance, Character, and The Bounds of Sense (II)" in *Raritan* 5 (3) (Winter 1986), 50.

9. James Dickey, "Angina," in *Poems: 1957–1967* (Middletown, Connecticut: Wesleyan University Press, 1967), 226–27.

10. James Dickey, "Buckdancer's Choice," in *Poems: 1957–1967*, 189–90.

11. Reg Saner, "Stroke," *The Georgia Review*, Spring 1984.

12. Bruce Weigl, "Anna's Grace," *The American Poetry Review*, 1990.

13. Alan Shapiro, "Someone Else," *The American Scholar*, Summer 1983.

14. John Mann Astrachan, "Jenny," in *Toward Solomon's Mountain: The Experience of Disability in Poetry*, Joseph L. Baird and Deborah S. Workman, eds. (Philadelphia: Temple University Press, 1986), 42.

15. Connie Bensley, "Waiting," *Times Literary Supplement*, September 11–17, 1987.

16. David Sweetman, "Mary," *Times Literary Supplement*, December 18–24, 1987.

17. Jack Coulehan, "The Knitted Glove," in *On Doctoring*, Richard Reynolds and John Stone, eds. (New York: Simon and Schuster, 1991), 374.

18. Peter Redgrove, "A Few Carats of Pain," *Times Literary Supplement*, March 20, 1987.

19. zana, "broken," in Baird and Workman, eds., *Toward Solomon's Mountain*, op. cit., 107.

20. Marilyn Davis, "Song for My Son," in Baird and Workman, eds., *Toward Solomon's Mountain*, 49.

21. Clara Claiborne Park, *The Siege* (Boston: Little, Brown, 1982), 160.

22. Ibid., 142.

23. Ibid., 163.

24. Arthur Frank, *At the Will of the Body* (Boston: Houghton Mifflin, 1991), 11.

25. Ibid., 26.

26. John Berger and Jean Mohr, *A Fortunate Man* (New York: Pantheon Books, 1967), 55.

27. Ibid., 69.

28. Ibid., 76.

29. Ibid.

30. Sallie Tisdale, *Harvest Moon: Portrait of a Nursing Home* (New York: Henry Holt, 1987), 144.

31. Ibid., 16.

32. See Charles Taylor, "The Politics of Recognition," in *Multiculturalism and "The Politics of Recognition,"* ed. Amy Gutmann (Princeton, N.J.: Princeton University Press, 1992), esp. 25: " . . . our identity is partly shaped by recognition or its absence, often by the misrecognition of others, and so a person or group of people can suffer real damage, real distortion, if the people or society around them mirror back to them a confining or demeaning or contemptible picture of themselves. Nonrecognition or misrecognition can inflict harm, can be a form of oppression, imprisoning someone in a false, distorted, and reduced mode of being."

33. Sallie Tisdale, *The Sorcerer's Apprentice: Tales of the Modern Hospital* (New York: McGraw-Hill, 1986), 8.

34. Berger and Mohr, *A Fortunate Man*, 134 and 78.

7

CHRONIC ILLNESS AND FREEDOM

GEORGE J. AGICH

GIVEN THE PROMINENCE of autonomy in medical ethics, it is important to explore its implications for chronic illness. Because the concept of autonomy itself is problematic, its application to chronic illness provides an important occasion for reassessing the meaning of autonomy in medical ethics.[1] Chronic illness offers an alternative model of illness to the standard acute care model that provides a paradigm for much medical ethics discourse. To see why this is the case requires a discussion of the assumptions associated with the concept of acute illness that support the liberal model of autonomy as well as of the ways that chronic illness deviates from this model. Highlighting these differences provides a format not only for questioning the adequacy of the standard model of autonomy, but for articulating a view of autonomy that supplements standard treatments without necessarily replacing autonomy with other principles. Admittedly, one could adopt a more radical approach and argue that the concept of autonomy itself should be consigned to the scrap heap, replacing it with a concept of beneficence or justice. Such an approach, however, is fundamentally wrongheaded, though to develop the reasons for rejecting it would only distract from the task at hand, namely, to try to make sense of the association of autonomy and chronic illness (Agich 1993).

The term *chronic illness* is quite ambiguous, though not more so than the notion of autonomy itself. Chronic illness functions as a Janus-like counterpart to the concept of acute illness, the main surface difference being the temporal duration and the prospect of recovery or cure. Chronic illness includes a set of conditions such as discomforts and disabilities ranging from morning pains from mild cases of arthritis to its crippling and degenerative forms; it includes both physical discomfort and disabilities and the psychological burdens of living with pain and disability. Chronic illness also includes conditions whose symptoms are virtually nonexistent or inconsequential for everyday life (depending on the kinds of activities engaged in), though the disease threatens an abrupt intrusion at every point, such as heart disease or some forms of epilepsy. Chronic illness also embraces diseases that specifically involve the effacement of personality or decisional capacity. Various degenerative diseases of the central nervous system, such as Alzheimer's, affect not only memory functions, but affective and cognitive functions as well. Given the wide array of diseases that satisfy the general features of chronic illness, it might be best to approach the question of the relationship of autonomy and chronic illness by focusing on the contrasting model of acute illness and the view of autonomy that dominates medical ethics.

Acute Illness

On one highly influential account, the sick person is someone who occupies a specific social role: *the sick role*. As described by Talcott Parsons, this role has four essential features: first, recovery from the incapacity is seen as being beyond the power of the individual person's own will; second, the incapacity is seen as a legitimate basis for an exemption from normal role and task responsibilities, hence the individual is not held accountable and is expected to surrender normal role responsibilities to others; third, the sick role is legitimated as a special social role, because the condition is both undesirable and entails the obligation that the person do everything necessary to get well; and fourth, since the natural course of events cannot be relied upon to improve the condition, the sick person is responsible for seeking out competent professional help (Parsons 1958: 428–479).

This model clearly supports professional over patient autonomy. The sick person suffers an episodic disability. Cure is reasonably expected and with it full resumption of normal social role responsibilities. The sick person undergoes a dramatic transformation on this model. In the first place, the sick person is no longer responsible for, even if actually able to carry out, normal activities. Passivity is thus a normative expectation, especially in terms of the prescribed deference to professional authority. The patient is literally a patient, that is, a (mostly) passive recipient of treatment. Patient autonomy on this model is thus an all-or-none proposition that is represented by two competing readings.

In one reading, patient autonomy is by definition waived or seriously compromised by illness (Pellegrino and Thomasma 1981; Daniels 1986). Because the patient is not fully an agent, the patient is vulnerable. This vulnerability is protected by the practitioner's concern for patient welfare (beneficence), which normatively guides all clinical decision making. This view accepts autonomy, but finding it absent in acute illness—as a matter of definition, not empirical determination, to be sure—professional authority is legitimated.

The legal doctrine of informed consent represents the other reading of the same situation. It regards this asymmetry of power and knowledge between patient and practitioner as a defect and regards the professional ethic of beneficence as paternalistic; as a corrective, it mandates disclosure of relevant risks and benefits of proposed treatments by the practitioner to redress the imbalance of knowledge. Disclosure of information evidently addresses only the imbalance of knowledge. This is all that is necessary since patients are regarded by defenders of patient autonomy as rational, free, competent decision makers. (As with the other position, this is a matter of definition, not empirical determination.) They possess all the relevant factors in deciding about treatment, such as their own beliefs and values, their own desires and preferences, except for technical information about the diagnosis, prognosis, and treatment. This deficiency is readily correctable by the disclosure requirement.

A number of simplifying assumptions underlie the acute care model of illness and the way that the principle of autonomy is relied upon to correct its deficiencies. Because illness is thought of as temporally discrete, the dominant concern is explicit decision making about, for example, diagnosis and treatment. It is thus easy to assume that patients only lack relevant knowledge or information but are otherwise competent agents. Needless to say, this model is hopelessly naive about the psychological state of patients needing medical care. By blithely assuming competence, the psychological aspects of illness and treatment are bypassed. Also, the model focuses exclusively on the relationship between the ill person and health professionals. In fact, the model requires a formal involvement with and deference to health professionals. The model kicks in, as it were, at the point where the sick person leaves the normal world of everyday life and enters the world of professional health care. As a result, the model is completely silent on the everyday aspects of illness and the relationship of autonomy thereto. This is not an insignificant omission. There are many other problems with this model of illness, but the most relevant for present purposes relate to the concept of autonomy that it seems to support.

The vulnerability of the acutely ill patient and the historically derived dominance of the physician foments tensions whose resolution is either complete deference to professional authority or insistence on autonomy-derived patient rights. The latter has been the common route of most bioethical work. The implicit model of autonomy on which the patient rights orientation relies, namely, a model of personal autonomy derived from political considerations, is particularly important. Given that the physician-patient relationship is perceived as a power struggle, it is natural that a political analogy is used. The political model of autonomy as independence is also a formidable cultural ideal, one that is expressed in the way various law courts and legislatures have erected an array of patient rights over recent decades. In light of the underlying model of acute illness, it is not surprising that a predominantly political paradigm has been central in medical ethical thought.

Autonomy

Treatment of autonomy in the medical ethics literature reflects cultural ideals in which personal autonomy is interpreted in predominantly legal-political terms. Although the concept as treated in the philosophical literature is frequently taken to involve a range of concerns (Christman 1988; 1989), the usual focus is on the the meaning of autonomy and not on the actual expressions of autonomy in every-day experience. Concern for the the concrete expressions of autonomy are usually restricted to classifying the general conditions under which individuals are able to make rational free choices. These conditions, for example, as expressed in the legal doctrine of informed consent, define a core set of concerns for medical ethics, though the tendency is that otherwise complicated conditions, such as disclosure of risks and benefits of treatment and its alternatives, comprehension of the information provided, the competence to consent, as well as the absence of coercive influence, are reduced to a simplifying formulation of clinical consent as an event rather than a process (Lidz, Appelbaum, and Meisel 1988).

Although autonomy is acknowledged by many authors to involve a family of meanings (Beauchamp and Childress 1983; Collopy 1986; 1988; Dworkin 1978; 1988; Thomasma 1984), it is usually expressed in terms that are congruent with the legal or political ideal of negative liberty, namely, the right to be left alone (Berlin 1969: 118–172). This ideal has been expressed under the banner of liberal political theory and is reflected in the prominent role that the language of patient rights enjoys in medical ethical discourse. The tendency in the medical ethics literature interestingly mirrors the tendency in political theory to eschew or at least avoid positive accounts of autonomy for fear that they inevitably involve dangerous authoritarian tendencies or unsupported and unsupportable metaphysical assumptions about the nature of the human good (Berlin 1969: 131, 135–141; Young 1896: 5). The underlying legal/political model of autonomy as negative freedom or freedom from restraint is central to liberal political theory and has had considerable influence in medical ethics (e.g., Engelhardt 1982), particularly through the concept of informed consent (Faden and Beauchamp 1986). Its importance and pervasiveness can hardly be overestimated.

In this view, personal autonomy prominently features the attributes and values of self-reliance, personal preference, and self-assertion. Self-reliance involves the capacity to provide for one's own needs without another's help. Personal preference focuses attention on the phenomena of choice and decision making, so that most treatments of autonomy focus on the absence of obstacles to choice (Bergmann 1977). Self-assertion points to the requirement that being free necessarily involves the active pursuit of the fulfillment of one's own desire. It is not enough to have desires or to make choices: one must be actively engaged in their accomplishment and fulfillment to be truly free on this view. So construed, autonomy involves a view of persons as isolated and independent rational and competent decision makers who are, by definition, involved in a ceaseless pursuit of the fulfillment of their own preferences, for without such pursuit and fulfillment, autonomy would be a vacuous concept on this view. Anything that thwarts the attainment of one's desires necessarily curtails freedom; as a result, noninterference becomes the overriding imperative.

Clearly, a model of illness that recognizes compromised ability and accepts its main features as ineliminable is strikingly discordant with this conception of the robustly autonomous person. Such a self is independent and self-sufficient, not dependent or burdened by anything like the range of symptoms and sufferings that comprise chronic illness. This is so perhaps less as a product of the strictly political source of the model than of its generally abstract character. Like so many ethical theories, the theory of patient autonomy in medical ethics relies on a rather abstract formulation of the nature of the physician-patient relationship, the context and circumstances of decision making, and the existential conditions of patienthood. In this way of viewing things, autonomy, too, is comfortably conceived as far removed from actual everyday circumstances. To remedy this signal defect, an analysis that attends to actual autonomy in the everyday world, rather than autonomy regarded under ideal conditions, is required (Agich 1990c; 1993: 76–113). Before discussing such an approach in terms of chronic illness, however, we need to be clear about the relationship of this analysis to some wider concerns about autonomy in ethical theory.

Although there are deficiencies associated with standard accounts of autonomy, there is good reason to defend the underlying liberal political theory precisely as a legal and political theory that defines important public and social values undergirding the meaning of liberal society. However, one can without contradiction criticize its unbridled extension beyond the legal/political realm into ethics (Larmore 1987). Recently, liberal theory has come under considerable attack by a motley set of thinkers under the banner of communitarianism (Bellah et al. 1985;

Hauerwas 1981; MacIntyre 1981; 1988; Perry 1988; Sandel 1982) on the ground that the liberal ideas of individualism and autonomy sever individuals from the cultural and historical traditions that persons need to sustain themselves as moral agents. When all is said and done, however, communitarianism founders on its rejection of any contextual justification of moral beliefs or actions (Larmore 1987: 27–35). Communitarians believe that the objectivity of a particular moral belief can be established only if our moral beliefs can be established *as a whole* by reference to some extramoral telos. Such a view is an epistemological foundationalism carried over into the realm of ethics (Larmore 1987: 29); the view commits most versions of communitarian thought to serious theoretical deficiencies. Given its stringent requirement for objectivity, it is no surprise that communitarianism has generally failed to establish such objectivity. Even so, the communitarian critique of the liberal ideas of individualism and autonomy as independence is quite apt. Thus, one can with good reason accept the core elements of this critique of individualism and autonomy as independence without rejecting liberal theory as such (Agich 1993).

It is quite defensible to argue that the deficiencies in the liberal view of autonomy for ethics can be acknowledged without committing oneself to an alternative foundationalist theory of the primacy of community or tradition while arguing that *actual autonomy* is an emergent phenomenon that necessarily involves individuals existing in interdependent socially and historically determined relationships. In other words, a main strand of the communitarian critique—that the liberal view of autonomy is ethically inadequate—can be accepted without wholly rejecting liberal theory. This point is important, because the question of the meaning of autonomy in chronic illness hinges on whether autonomy is a relevantly central ethical concept. Communitarian thought, like beneficence-centered approaches,[2] simply fails to give autonomy its due. For this reason, I bypass these alternatives.

Despite its limitations as a full account of autonomy, the liberal view of autonomy as independence does have important implications for chronic illness. In the first and more obvious sense, liberal principles imply that individuals who are chronically ill are responsible for their own decisions. Chronically ill individuals are presumed to be able to make decisions for themselves. On the basis of this (rebuttable) presumption a bulwark of protection for chronically ill persons can be established. As is well recognized, autonomy supports the language of rights, rights that provide individuals with an insulating and protecting shell (Glendon 1991; Ladd 1978; Wellman 1985). Such rights protect individuals from the intrusive, albeit sometimes benevolent, actions of others. Reflection on freedom in this first sense, then, implies the articulation of a panoply of rights.

To respect autonomy on the liberal model is to accord patients a range of rights as a foundation for protecting their moral status. What is most relevant is that the patient be regarded as agent, not simply as patient (MacIntyre 1977). While that implication is important, it does not take us very far unless we can provide a fuller sense of what it means to be an agent in the everyday world. Insisting on the rights of patients does, to be sure, help us to understand that chronic illness, like acute illness, involves situations in which patients are vulnerable. The protection of this vulnerability from unwarranted intrusion is usefully secured by the fundamental right to noninterference, a right that expresses the central ideal of autonomy as negative freedom. Much could (and perhaps should) be said about the applicability of various rights in specific kinds of chronic illness, for example, rights protecting the disabled from various kinds of discrimination, or the right to an obstacle-free environment for those with physical handicaps, but I leave that task for others, not because these are ethically nugatory matters, but because they are such standard implications of the mainstream view of autonomy. My concern runs in a different direction, a direction that crosses the mainstream. I want to explore the territory latent behind the ideal of autonomy as independence and chart some of its watershed.

The Patient as Ideally Autonomous

One main problem with most liberal-inspired treatments of autonomy is the inadequacy of the underlying political model, namely, state sovereignty, for understanding the autonomy of persons. On this model, the person is understood on analogy with an ideal autonomous political unit that has independence from the laws and governance of other states. To be autonomous in this sense is to be sovereign (to have unfettered authority or power) within a specific political domain. Many naturally think that the autonomy of individuals analogously involves independence from the authority of others. As a result, autonomy is defined privatively as negative freedom in terms of the absence of coercion or the absence of dependence (Berlin 1969: 122; Young 1986: 3).

This model of political autonomy can be shown to be defective since various conditions, including economic underdevelopment, can make it impossible even for states to control their own destinies in meaningful ways, though they continue to make and administer their own laws (Young 1986: 7). Even at the level of the state, this model is somewhat simplistic. Nonetheless, it has played an important role in various articulations of personal autonomy, including the conception of negative liberty articulated by Isaiah Berlin (1969: 122), namely, that to be at liberty is to be unobstructed by others. It finds expression in various accounts of rights as defining spheres of activities in which interference by others is similarly illegitimate (Richards 1981; Wellman 1985: 102).

Economic and various other conditions, of course, restrict the options open to individuals and so necessarily restrict their liberty in important ways (Feinberg 1978). Most thinkers do not much worry about these conditions, regarding them as empirical complications of the theory. Such restrictions, however, do seem to be an essential fact of life. They are unavoidable aspects of actual autonomy and so need to be taken seriously in any account of the relationship of autonomy and chronic illness. That these conditions tend to be overlooked in many treatments of autonomy should caution us regarding the degree to which we should rely upon such an orientation. In fact, in the context of long-term care of elders I have argued for the primacy of actual autonomy over abstract theoretical conceptions (Agich 1990c; 1993). Actual autonomy focuses not only on the everyday detail in cases of conflict and circumstances of choice, but on the structural aspects of the experience of the agent as autonomous.

One dominant focus of standard accounts of autonomy is on choice. To be free is to have unfettered and unrestricted choice from a given range of options or alternatives. What is crucial is that there are alternatives and that one's choice of alternatives is not constrained in any way. Clearly, this model is simplistic. Individuals can be afforded choices that are themselves intolerable or burdensome. The absence of constraint hardly makes being confronted by unbearable choice a positive matter. The tragic aspect of choice is not readily accommodated by the standard model. Yet, the everyday experiences of an individual suffering chronic illness inevitably involve various compromises, compromises that, though freely chosen (in that they are unconstrained by "others"), are constrained by the very nature of the illness itself. No wonder, then, that illness gets personified, as something *Other*. The concept of the Other serves both the psychological and the cultural tendency to regard anything that threatens our sense of self as alien (Gilman 1988), but it also integrates the experience of chronic illness into the comfortable framework of the liberal account of autonomy as choice. Since the illness is Other, *it* constrains my choice; in doing so, *it* excuses me from accountability.

This model of choice, however, is too removed from actual conditions of experience to be very useful. Another model is needed, one that focuses on actual, as opposed to ideal, autonomy. Rather than a metaphor of a road or path with alternatives branching therefrom, one might think of choice as a component of action in the social world. The alternative metaphor that might appropriately capture this would be that of crossing a field of grass. As in the earlier metaphor, there is movement and a terminus, but the appearance of a fixed structure is gone and actual choice becomes a diffuse feature in a wider set of phenomena. Depending on where one entered the field or one's interests, purposes, or needs, one might follow the natural gradient of the field, as in a leisurely stroll, or let it work against one, as an avid runner might do to build stamina. Certainly, the field might be crisscrossed with paths from previous travelers, but they will only be evident in the irregularities in the growing patterns of the grass, its deviation from the perpendicular, but not as a smooth predefined way. The influences of others and society will also be marked out as patterns or tendencies, not causally-determining forces or logically clear alternatives. One might, of course, note the various ways in advance and choose the one that appeared to afford the least resistance or moved in the "right" direction, but the metaphor does not require that action and choice be so structured to be regarded as autonomous. There is considerably more room for the actual exercise of autonomy creatively and individually to make its own way across the field of life. A person's action might be guided by the evident patterns marked out in the field, but they might be guided as well by literally loftier objectives, because one followed the flight of a grouse without care for the field itself or simply ambled in a general direction or toward a specific endpoint, such as a particular tree at the end of the field. How the transit of the field is interpreted will thus reflect various purposes and interests, none of which are priviledged over another by the model's structure.

The metaphor of the field of grass is far more adequate for the purposes of understanding the relation of autonomy and chronic illness. No longer can we restrict our attention to idealized cases of decision making under hypothetical conditions in which agents are assumed to be fully rational and competent, able to clearly see through to the consequences of their choices, and capable of reflective deliberation. Such a model, to be sure, plays an important role in legal and political theory, but it proves rather inadequate for grasping the complex reality of actual autonomy. Actual autonomy is not best understood in terms of decisional nodes, but in the daily ebb and flow of action and experience.

Actual Autonomy and Chronic Illness

While an acute illness befalls an individual, and so an individual literally suffers or undergoes it, chronic illness involves suffering as a specific mode of existence. One endures in the face of chronic illness, with chronic illness, or as chronically ill. Each of these modifiers indicates a phenomenologically distinctive experience of chronic illness. To be chronically ill one does not need to be a patient. Chronic illness need not be severely incapacitating, and even when it is, the individual is only episodically, if at all, a patient wholly in the hands of a health professional. The chronic, perduring character of chronic illness complicates the person's adoption of the sick role. The sick role requirement that one surrender one's normal social role responsibilities entails not just a brief loss of freedom as the price of cure, but a potential compromising of one's own identity in the case of chronic illness. There is good reason to argue that identity is prior to freedom, because to be free means that one has an established identity or set of identifications that define the self as its *own* self. Without such an identity, action and autonomy would be mere idealizations without substantial content. In the chronically ill the orientation necessarily shifts from removal of the cause of suffering to the suffering itself, since the suffering affects the core identity of the self.

The incapacities and disabilities, the experiences of pain or various symptoms, are not themselves signs of something wrong that has befallen the individual, but rather are of a kind of life that the individual must live. Living with chronic illness thus necessarily means suffering an alteration in who one is. Suffering, unfortunately, is not something that in itself sustains value. Indeed, the standard concept of autonomy implies a robust independent individual capable of acting without help and in the face of the onslaught of the world. Given this dominant cultural ideal, to be chronically ill means that one has to endure an additional disvalue and burden, namely, that of giving living testimony to the incompleteness, if not falsity, of basic cultural values. It is no wonder, then, that there are movements insisting on the rights of the disabled and other individuals suffering from chronic illness to full participation in society. Though their capacities may be limited by disease, autonomy can be respected by according them rights, for example, to an environment free of obstacles to full employment and to access to various social services. I have no interest in critically analyzing these movements, but only observe that they make sense against a background in which the very experience of incapacity and disability is a surd element, an element that cannot be accepted, because it is incapable of being reconciled with the robust sense of abstract autonomy that dominates our cultural attitudes and beliefs.

There is frequently talk about "managing" chronic illness. Although it is typically used in a professional sense, it does have other relevant associations. With the chronically ill patient, managing the illness is coincident with managing one's life. That is, the illness does not exist as some independent thing to be managed, but as an element or factor in a common negotiation with the world. This means that chronic illness involves a suffering that is far more subtle and pervasive than merely being made passive by an episode of acute illness.

Chronic illness thus invites reflection along a different axis, one that is all too infrequently attended to in the mainstream accounts deriving from liberal political theory. This axis is complementary to liberal theory, not inimical to it (Agich 1993: 13–46). Rather than focus on discrete choices and conflicts or dilemmas, chronic illness invites analysis of the mundane or interstitial features of action and experience in the social world. Attending to chronic illness helps us expand the understanding of autonomy in ways that are both exciting and important for medical ethics. In chronic illness, one undergoes the illness not as an intrusion into one's life, but as a way of life. Authors as diverse as Stewart Wolf (1961) and Thomas Mann (1967) have seen illness in this light. Chronic illness thus serves to shake us loose from the grip of the myth of acute illness, a myth that illness is essentially episodic and a transient intrusion into our lives, that illness is something that can always be cured and that normal functioning can be restored if only we would surrender ourselves to the miracles of modern medicine. Rather, chronic illness reminds us of our finitude and that our everyday lives involve inescapable compromise. This does not diminish the unique suffering of those who endure specific chronic diseases, but rather reminds us that to understand chronic illness is not like visiting some quaint countryside for a long weekend, but rather is an exercise that helps us gain a new perspective on the hustle and bustle of our own everyday lives.

Saying this leaves to one side the important phenomenological treatment of various kinds of chronic illness. My concern is primarily to develop an argument for a phenomenology and to make clear its significance for contemporary treatments of autonomy in medicine, not to describe any specific kind of chronic illness. Adopting this tack, of course, in no way denies that the distinctive phenomenological features of chronic illness are ethically relevant or that they need to be considered in the everyday dealings with chronic illness. For present purposes, I simply offer a more coarse-grained account. Since chronic illness is such a motley class, I confine my discussion to two general features that indicate the way that autonomy and chronic illness are interrelated in the social world of everyday life: temporality and affectivity.

Temporality

Humans are essentially temporal; they come into being and develop as persons in time and constitute their identities historically. They develop and express themselves as persons only through their participation in a social world. Thus, relationships with others are necessary both for a sense of self and for a sense of world. To interpret autonomy properly one must consider the temporal aspect of human existence not simply as a frame for choice or decision making, but as an existential and social matrix against which the very conception of something as a project is possible (Schutz 1970: 67–96).

The notion that there is an objective time "out there" is itself a feature of the everyday world. Although we act as if time existed objectively, it is a feature of the shared world of experience. Shared time helps define not only the social world of action and work, but also a fundamental orientation for the self. In the social world, individuals go about the myriad activities that comprise their day-to-day existence. Events that significantly modify that existence, for example, illness or a special event such as a marriage, a holiday, or the death of a friend or loved one, affect the perception of time itself. As a result, the typical ebb and flow of events is perceptually deformed and shaped by the significance of the events.

Chronic illness, too, has an effect on temporal experience. The temporal nature of a chronic illness consists not only in its persistence over time, but in its effect on the temporal structure of the experience of the self and others. To be able to act and to gear into the world requires an experienced temporal relationship between my choice or decision to act, the action, and the outcome. The pain or disability associated with some forms of chronic illness distort this relationship. This can be seen by reflecting on the applicability of the distinction between decisional and executional autonomy (Collopy 1988).

In extreme cases, a severely disabled person might still be able to decide for herself (decisional autonomy is intact, in other words), yet unable to carry out her actions without assistance. The impairment in executional autonomy not only makes the person unfree, but affects her experience of herself as agent. Providing enabling assistance, such as transportation, shopping, or housework, can enhance the autonomy of the chronically ill person. Even so, the distortion in the person's self-perception of her agency, expressed in feelings of frustration and helplessness is partly associated with the way that our sense of agency depends on a temporally experienced relationship between choice, action, and outcome.

In their day-to-day lives people are usually busy with many things, and many interests compete for their attention (Zerubavel 1979; 1981). Alterations in daily schedules or routines either slow down or speed up the sense of passing time and give experience a heavy or a light feeling. The qualitative aspects of the flow of time are affected likewise by the symptoms, disabilities, and incapacities associated with chronic illnesses. Time is the universal medium of experience, but it is not a neutral medium. It carries associations and meanings that themselves influence experience. For example, limitations in habitual actions created by newly incurred disabilities entail a need for adaptation. Time can hang heavy for one newly unable to do things for herself. Individuals used to free movement are burdened not just by the obstacles they confront when wheelchair-bound, but by the need to accommodate to the increased time required for even routine, everyday tasks.

When someone says they do not have time for something, they deny that thing its relative importance or value. When they make time for something, they focus attention on it, and so thereby value that thing. A child or spouse who complains that the father who works constantly does not have time for her is complaining that she feels devalued by the father's inattention or preoccupation with other things, even while the father might actually spend time in her presence. The child or spouse may complain that the father is not really *here* in the very time purportedly spent together! Time spent with the preoccupied father goes too quickly or does not afford a sense of openness, because it seems that preoccupation intrudes not only on the details of the experienced but on its temporal quality as well.

A chronically ill person might employ various techniques to solicit attention designed to bring significant others into her temporal world, as a ploy to have them make time for herself not simply as a patient needing professional or technical care but as a person needing the attention of other humans. In this regard, it is important to distinguish the tasks performed or services rendered from care that is manifested with concern. One can adequately provide a service without due regard for the person receiving it, without affective or emotional engagement, but care necessarily requires engagement and engagement involves people tuning into one another's temporal stream, as Alfred Schutz termed it, "making music together":

> It appears that all possible communication presupposes a mutual tuning-in relationship between the communicator and the addressee of the communication. This relationship is established by the reciprocal sharing of the Other's flux of experiences in inner time, by living through a vivid present together, by experiencing this togetherness as a "We." Only within this experience does the Other's conduct become meaningful to the partner tuned in on him—that is, the Other's body and its movements can be and are interpreted as a field of expression of events within his inner life. . . . Communicating with one another presupposes, therefore, the simultaneous partaking of the partners in various dimensions of outer and inner time—in short in growing older together. This seems to be valid for all kinds of communication. (1971b: 177–78)

If this observation is correct, then the importance of time in establishing a common and shared world and in making possible genuine communication becomes apparent. This is, however, a double-edged problem. Not only is the chronically ill person's experience of time affected, but so is that of others. Adapting one's usual pace to someone who is hobbled with pain creates a shared temporal burden for them both. This can either be an occasion for significant, though unremarkable, caring or an occasion for anger and frustration. The whole point of talking about actual autonomy is to have a way to conceptualize a concrete historically and socially determined self. Hence, it helps us understand why the effect of chronic illness on significant others can affect the true autonomy of the affected person.

Chronic illness affects relations with others in myriad ways. Bonds of affection and commitment are not established all at once or by logical definition, but through time. These bonds are temporally constituted, not in terms of some future benefit, some rational decision regarding what is appropriate or best in a given set of circumstances, but on the basis of what is felt or judged to be "right," "proper," or "appropriate" based on who we are. Who one is is based on who one became in the past, and the past is always a shared past. The past exerts an important, but not a deterministic influence on all of us. It gives a basis and a foundation for movement into the uncertainty of the future. On its basis, each of us develops a plethora of skills, recipes for action or what sociologists call typifications, namely, generalized expectations that structure our experiences and enable us to function in the social world. Included with these typifications are emotional bonds or beliefs that involve the trust (or mistrust) that individuals have in one another and in their own abilities. One signal problem with the liberal model of autonomy is that it assumes that individuals are isolated and independent. They exist in an atemporal "eternal now" contemplating the implications and consequences of their actions in an idealized future. But to experience options as choices is not some conceptual or logical exercise. Choices are experienced as choices insofar as they are meaningful options for an individual, as they cohere with patterns of expectation developed in the past.

The human mind cannot function if it is overwhelmed by options whose variety is so great or whose novelty cannot be readily assimilated into the person's frame of reference. For the chronically ill, the relevant frame of reference is on typical experience, experience structured in terms of mundane matters that the rest of us simply take for granted. We assume without reflection that we will awake refreshed and without pain, yet such an expectation may not be reasonable for the person suffering from arthritis. Arthritic pain sets a limit on the day even before daily life has been resumed, and it threatens throughout daily activities to cut short, interrupt, or otherwise distort experiences and events. Effort is required to prepare for activities or their sometimes painful sequelae. For the rest of us, activity or inactivity is mostly a matter of indifference. For the arthritic, however, daily life is affected by the constant presence or promise of pain that sets temporal limits on activities. Medications and other treatments also impose temporal demands. Some medications need to be taken with meals or have untoward side effects that constantly need to be considered by the chronically ill person; other treatments need to be scheduled or take time to complete. Every significant action or alteration in pattern, therefore, entails the need to reassess the temporal context. If a medication causes drowsiness, then one has to plan for a limited time of full alertness before the inevitable side effect occurs and blunts one's functional attentiveness.

Because chronic illness is illness that extends into the future, it defines the present from the future and in light of the pain, the disability, and ultimately the death that it portends. One crucial concern, therefore, is the meaning and function of hope. Individuals suffering from chronic illness, by definition, cannot by mere exercise of will or professional ministration change the basic nature of their condition. To try only breeds despair. Defenders of the mainstream model of autonomy often forget this compelling point. By underscoring and stressing choice in a circumstance in which some of the most meaningful options are simply unavailable, they recommend what seems either absurd or cruel. Unfortunately, when this is recognized, the only recourse on this view is to talk of hopelessness. *Hopelessness* is a term frequently used by physicians to mean that no effective treatment is available or that cure is impossible. For modern medicine, relying as it does on the acute care paradigm, hope implies effective treatment. If there is no effective treatment, no prospect of cure, and no return to normality, then there is no hope. If that is the case, then the ultimate condition of everyone is hopeless. We are all going to die. But is hope properly conceptualized in terms of ability to effect cure? Doctors and health professionals frequently advocate interventions and procedures long after their purpose has expired. When queried they respond that to withdraw treatment or even to discuss its removal would be to take away all hope. This is a rather unfortunate understanding of the meaning of hope.

The concept of hope does not require such a restricted understanding; it need not be restricted to a technological fix. Rather, hope is a virtue defining one's bearing toward the future. To hope is not to expect, much less demand, a "good" or "acceptable" outcome, but to experience forthrightly and with fortitude whatever comes one's way. A person without hope is literally a non-person, since hope is required for a person to face autonomously even the most dire future. The opposite of hope, despair, is correlatively not a matter of mere subjective feeling, but a matter of the bearing of the individual toward the future. With hope the individual is attached to and nurtured by others, whereas in despair, one is alone and abandoned. The irony of physicians' speaking of hopeless cases is the failure to see that hope persists not in technological fixes but in the emotional support and care that the sick receive. In the case of the chronically ill patient, *care* and *taking care* in the course of routine and typical everyday interactions are sometimes hard to differentiate. Due regard for a chronically ill individual as a person in the normal flow of events and shared experiences, such as putting up with their attention to their bodily processes or allowing them to be dependent, may be more important than providing any special kind of service-defined care.

Affectivity

Persons develop and change through feeling. One important way that this occurs involves the claims that feeling places on individuals. Affectivity connects or separates individuals one from another. The relation to significant others is not extrinsic, but is integral to the sense of one's self. This commitment is mostly prereflective, preceding and mostly preempting calculation of its costs.

Commitment to a chronically ill person, like a parent's commitment to the child, is usually forged in the continuity of time, not predicated on any particular episode or event. Hence, one does not so much choose, but finds oneself committed. This explains the sense that spouses or children experience when confronted with a loved one who becomes chronically ill; they are stuck without the benefit of choice. It would be a gross mistake to say that a loving parent or spouse chose the chronic illness for another or chose the role of caregiver or observer of the suffering. Rather than choosing, one can affirm or deny the illness and in so doing affirm or deny the value of the person suffering it, but one does not choose the illness itself. Autonomy is thus revealed less in the exercise of choice than in a personal commitment that is either affirmed or rejected. The apparent frequency with which individuals in our society affirm commitments to those with chronic illness shows how strong the affective bonds forged in the continuity of relationships are and the important way that recognizing and respecting one's responsibilities comprises who we are as autonomous agents.

The importance of affectivity for the ethics of chronic illness is thus connected to traditional concepts of character, namely, those distinctive dispositions that comprise the basic nature of moral personhood. It is important in this regard to distinguish an *occurrent* sense of autonomy, the sense that is intended when we speak of people acting autonomously in a particular circumstance or situation, and a comprehensive or *dispositional* sense of autonomy that defines the overall course of a person's life. Only this dispositional or comprehensive sense of autonomy allows an individual to enjoy a life that is unified, orderly, and free from self-defeating conflict over fundamental beliefs and values (Young 1986: 8). Such a dispositional sense of autonomy is possible only because the self is affectively related to itself and to others. Affectivity provides the glue, as it were, that joins the various episodes and pieces of one's life into a coherent whole. Chronic illness surely subjects this glue to a daily test of its adhesiveness.

Action manifests the basic spontaneity of human life, the autonomy of persons. Action, however, is not simply a matter of choosing a course of action, but involves "gearing into" the world, actually engaging in physical work in and on the world. Through effort and feeling we experience the world and others. People feel rather than think the world, yet the main ways of conceptualizing autonomy all stress the cognitive and decisional aspects rather than the affective or dispositional. As a consequence, an important range of considerations are excluded.

Daydreaming, wondering, and fantasy of various sorts, including wishing or reminiscence, involve modifications of our basic orientation to the world. These modifications provide us with the experiential depth and embellishment that persons savor. Such activities remake the world by forming new meanings and interpretations. Indeed, such ability is tied up with the basic sense of an individual as a spontaneous or autonomous conscious subject and does not usually impair or conflict with an individual's ability to attend sufficiently to practicalities of the everyday world. As a matter of fact, we manage in the everyday world because we are able to segregate and segment our experience into various "finite provinces of meaning" (Schutz 1971a: 207–259, 340–347). Movement from one finite province of meaning to another, especially to the finite province that has been termed the "paramount reality" or the world of everyday shared social experience, involves effort and the experience of shock in transitioning from the world of imagination or memory, for example, back to the world of daily life and work. Associated with these various provinces of meaning or worlds are specific feelings and moods that make these worlds hospitable or foreboding, comfortable or uncomfortable, familiar or strange (Bachelard 1969). These feelings infuse the everyday world with its textures of meaning and provide motivations for moving from one realm of meaning to another.

Chronic illness might be constructively regarded in these terms. What, for example is required of the diabetic or the person suffering from renal disease or colitis for whom eating and drinking become matters of great concern and are reconceived by health providers in terms of fluid and food intake, of prescribed and proscribed items? Asthmatics or people with food allergies must constantly monitor and be aware of environmental factors or food ingredients lest contact prompt an allergic response of wheezing, difficulty in breathing, hives, or anaphylaxis. For such a person the world is a place of eminent and imminent danger. Hence, the attunement to self that normally characterizes autonomous agents is turned around in these chronically ill patients into a needful attention to the environment. Like a cat on the prowl, for whom every movement solicits an attentive response, chronically ill persons, too, can be drawn outside themselves to an environment that poses danger not opportunity. This environment includes not only the ambient world, but the patient's own body that can acquire an alien presence. Like the animal, the chronically ill patient must live outside himself rather than, as we normally are in everyday life, immersed in the activities themselves. Even when the illness involves subjective experiences, such as pain, the self is drawn away from its involvement in normal activity and is reflexively drawn back upon itself in order to maintain a reasonable state of equilibrium. Understandably, then, the fundamental anxiety that structures everyday existence and explains our actions in the social world is given a focus and prominence in an illness that cannot be readily set aside in daily projects and activities.[3] For this reason, chronically ill persons can appear to be preoccupied with self when in fact they are actually preoccupied with experiences that are alien to the self, that intrude on the self in everyday life and demand attention in their own right.

Under these circumstances, individuals necessarily retreat from the everyday world to other "worlds" or provinces of meaning. When the illness and symptoms are severe, the orientation to the world of everyday life, if not loosened, is altered in various ways and so the energies of the self are understandably directed away from routine activities and toward the general task of constituting new structures of meaning. Coping strategies, in effect, involve utilizing or developing techniques to ameliorate the disengagement from the everyday world that chronic illness foists on persons. To cope is to function in the face of adversity and suffering, and the need to cope underscores how central the social world of everyday life is to our very existence as human persons, and the central role of feeling in the experience.

At the basis of our existence as autonomous agents is an affective experience not of ourselves as decision makers, as individuals capable of rational choice, but as finite beings with desires and needs (Haworth 1986). In everyday life this experience is suppressed, hidden like the framework of a house within the ceilings, floors, and walls of our projects and plans. The primary nature of actual autonomy cannot be adequately understood if affectivity is left unconsidered. Attention to affectivity comparable to that accorded to cognition and will in standard accounts of autonomy as free choice is at least required, because it is not the choice or decision that defines the action so much as it is the felt experience of it both as my own and as the embodiment of a purposive intention (Zaner 1981: 42–43).

Through kinesthetic feelings, the human person becomes present to herself and at the same time presents the self to others in the world in embodied action. Bodily action thus enacts the self in the world in a way that simultaneously reveals the self to the person and the world. That is why our experiences and our actions are always ambiguous, always uncertain, both to ourselves and to others. Individuals experience themselves and the world not only through bodily feelings of mobility or immobility, but also through the experience of space and time as heavy or light, open or closed, light or dark, happy or sad, and so forth through a veritable infinity of possibilities. As affective and sentient entities, persons exist in dynamic tension with the world and with others.

Chronic, unlike acute, illness does not involve a disengagement from this common world of experience, but is more a way of experiencing the world under specific conditions of disability, incapacity, or pain. It is an experiencing of the world not as a robustly free self isolated and independent from others, but as dependent and vulnerable. In an important sense, chronic illness, far more than even the high drama of acute life-threatening conditions, reveals that to be actually, as opposed to ideally, autonomous is to live an essentially compromised existence under contingent conditions. Actually autonomous persons thus are not neutrally situated decision makers rationally and disinterestedly calculating the costs and benefits of various alternatives. Rather, alternatives or choices impinge upon them in preformed and predetermined or typified patterns, patterns that are experienced meaningfully through the vivid colors of emotion and mood and not the black and white of quantitative calculation. In a sense, the world and other persons are experienced not as nouns, but adjectivally, that is, as colored by emotion and feelings.

Frequently individuals who are chronically ill complain of fatigue. To feel tired is obviously an accompanying symptom of certain illnesses or a side effect of certain kinds of medication, but fatigue as an affective experience of the world is something altogether different. Institutional fatigue, for example, is clearly identifiable: a dull, slow motor activity, shuffling walk, slow arm movements, head bowed low, stooped shoulders, a gaze devoid of usual intensity, a desire to sit almost immediately after standing or to return to bed when one is forced to leave it. Institutionalized patients are typically more weary than the existing conditions seem to warrant. Fatigue is best understood by regarding it as a peculiar kind of affective, subjective way of living through "something" rather than by examining the behavioral manifestations in isolation from the person who manifests them.

The main question is whether fatigue is best understood in terms of physiologically measurable alterations in muscle strength, which, among other things, can be noted by increased levels of lactic acid, or does it have to do, instead, with feelings occurring independent of the physiological conditions of muscle strength? Or, does it involve both?

The character of this problem is quite analogous to the problem of pain, owing to the similarities in the questions about the role of physiological functions in what appears to be a unique kind of subjective experience. It may be that complaints about fatigue and fatigue-related behaviors represent efforts to communicate something other than what we normally construe fatigue to mean (Bergsma and Thomasma 1982: 136–137). Failure to consider this alternative necessarily preempts the question of the meaning of this experience in the context of the life plan and life story of the chronically ill person as a developed self with formed identifications. Actual autonomy is thus bypassed because the complaints of fatigue seem unrelated to choice or will except as problems or obstacles to be removed. When the affective character of fatigue or other symptoms is bypassed, however, the concrete identity of the suffering self is also bypassed. What is true for fatigue might also be said for the myriad other symptoms that persons with chronic illnesses experience.

Conclusion

These brief observations regarding affectivity and temporality bear directly on the meaning of autonomy in chronic illness. Illness and impairment are circumstances that block one's typical or usual path or pattern of behavior in the world. In illness, whether acute or chronic, one's bodily enactment fails; hence, one's sense of personal identity is imperiled, because our identity is so intimately bound up with our embodiment. Even routine action becomes effortful; engaging in activities of daily living is burdensome and wearisome. A healthy person is relatively buoyant and free-floating in the course of his or her action in the world; illness, however, weighs one down and frequently manifests itself as lethargy or lassitude. As a result, the entire shape and texture of the world as experienced is altered for the ill person.

In chronic illness being ill permeates everyday experience. There is no time off for being sick. Sickness is infrequently a socially defined way of life for those who are chronically ill; except for those who adopt the sick role and assume patienthood, chronic illness comes with little social role guidance. For the chronically ill there is no clearly defined and socially sanctioned role analogous to the sick role.

Roles such as the disabled, the retarded, or the developmentally disabled are historically conditioned reactions to certain classes of chronically ill persons, but are not positive social roles. None of these illustrate in any helpful way the core meaning of autonomy in chronic illness. For these well-recognized class of persons, however, one can aptly appeal to the standard models of autonomy and insist on their rights to nondiscrimination and freedom of access, for example, but these classes neither exhaust the range of chronic illness nor explain the actual autonomy of the concrete suffering selves.

Consider the simple case of a person who develops heart disease and suffers angina. Previously, she functioned with relative independence and self-confidence. When angina occurs, the whole world is dramatically transformed and placed into question. At virtually any moment the searing pain might sound off like some hidden alarm warning of limits that cannot be breached, warning of the inescapable fact of death. New concerns become relevant, such as which physical activities are tolerable and which are not. Stairs, for example, now seem to have changed their proportion. The angina thus calls into question typical and taken-for-granted experiences of the world and the person's place therein. It presents problems in terms of relations with others, such as spouse and children, whose loving concern may itself threaten one's fundamental sense of self-worth. It would be a mistake to argue that the issues posed here are issues of independence, though independence is certainly one of the values at stake.

In circumstances like the one outlined above, the sometimes extensive and serious modifications of lifestyle that are necessary adaptations force the ill person to define herself in a new and different fashion. Doing so necessarily involves effort. Such effort is a signal and fundamental feature of what it means to be an autonomous person or self (Haworth 1986; Zaner 1981: 169). Accompanying this effort, no matter how feeble, maladaptive, or ineffective it may appear, are corollary experiences of anger, frustration, loss, and the myriad emotional reactions associated with physical illness and suffering. Understanding and dealing with these experiences serves both to provide the occasion for reestablishing the connection of the ill person with the social world and to provide the only sure location from which to care for those suffering from chronic illnesses.

The ethical problems posed by chronic illness are rather less dramatic and conflictual than those raised by the acute illness model. Chronic illness prompts analysis along a different and much neglected axis or dimension. Rather than consideration of conflicts and rights, chronic illness prompts consideration of the very nature of mundane experience and existence. It is here, in the middle of things, between the nodes of decision and conflict, that the true nature of autonomy emerges. The ethics of chronic illness is an ethics of the everyday, a set of concerns that unfortunately have been relegated to the periphery as bioethics adopted uncritically a legal/political paradigm. However, chronic illness does not itself recommend alternatives to liberal theory. The debate between communitarian, virtue-or character-based ethics and liberal-inspired accounts is quite frankly far too removed from the actuality of autonomy and the concrete reality of chronic illness to clarify the matter.

The true significance of chronic illness for medical ethics is the unique way that considerations such as whether persons are better conceived as isolated, rational, and free decision makers or as historically and socially dependent selves are brought into view. These considerations point less to conclusions about the nature of authority in society, as so many advocates of communitarianism and liberalism would like, than to the practical problems of living and experiencing the shared world under conditions of compromise and contingency. The nature of affective experience, of caring, and of caregiving relationships becomes more crucial than concern for the foundation of authority in ethical matters. The implications of these points admittedly bear on wider concerns about the nature of ethical theory and medical ethics, but the most important function of chronic illness is the way that it revises our standard assumptions about the nature of autonomy. Once we take chronic illness seriously, the complexity of actual expressions of autonomy is less likely to be eliminated from medical ethics by the operation of abstract analytical concepts.

NOTES

1. Long-term care of elders provides another fruitful context for critically reflecting on the meaning of autonomy; see Agich 1990c and 1993.

2. For a critical discussion of the appeal to beneficence in the debate over reform of the financing of health care, see Agich 1987; 1990a; 1990b.

3. An affective experience underlies the basic orientation of the agent in the world of everyday life; it was termed the *fundamental anxiety* by Alfred Schutz (1971a: 228). The entire system of relevances that governs us within the everyday natural attitude is founded on a basic experience of each individual, namely, I know that I shall die and I fear to die. This basic experience is the primordial anticipation from which all other experience originates. From the fundamental anxiety springs the many interrelated systems of hopes and fears, wants and satisfactions, chances and risks that incite persons within the everyday world to attempt mastery, overcome obstacles, and effortfully strive to realize projects and plans. The fundamental anxiety itself is a corollary of our existence as human beings

within the paramount reality of daily life: therefore, everyday hopes and fears and their correlated satisfactions and disappointments are grounded upon and only possible within the ambient social world of everyday life.

BIBLIOGRAPHY

Agich, George J. 1987. "Incentives and Obligations under Prospective Payment." *Journal of Medicine and Philosophy* 11: 123–144.

———. 1990a. "Medicine as Business and Profession." *Theoretical Medicine* 11: 311–324.

———. 1990b. "Rationing and Professional Autonomy." *Law, Medicine & Health Care* 18 (Spring-Summer): 77–84.

———. 1990c. "Reassessing Autonomy in Long-Term Care." *Hastings Center Report* 20 (6): 12–17.

———. 1993. *Autonomy and Long Term Care.* New York: Oxford University Press.

Bachelard, Gaston. 1969. *The Poetics of Space.* Maria Jolas, trans. Boston: Beacon Press.

Beauchamp, Tom L., and James F. Childress. 1983. *Principles of Biomedical Ethics*, Second Edition. New York and Oxford: Oxford University Press.

Bellah, Robert N., Richard Madsen, William N. Sullivan, Ann Swindler, and Steven M. Tipton. 1985. *Habits of the Heart: Individualism and Commitment in American Life.* Berkeley, CA: University of California Press.

Bergmann, Frithjof. 1977. *On Being Free.* Notre Dame, IN: University of Notre Dame Press.

Bergsma, Jurrit, and David Thomasma. 1982. *Health Care: Its Psychosocial Dimensions.* Pittsburgh, PA: Duquesne University Press.

Berlin, Isaiah. 1969. *Four Essays on Liberty.* Oxford: Oxford University Press.

Christman, John. 1988. "Constructing The Inner Citadel: Recent Work on The Concept of Autonomy." *Ethics* 99 (October): 109–124.

———., ed. 1989. *The Inner Citadel: Essays on Individual Autonomy.* New York and Oxford: Oxford University Press.

Collopy, Bart J. 1986. *The Conceptually Problematic Status of Autonomy.* Unpublished study prepared for The Retirement Research Foundation.

———. 1988. "Autonomy and Long Term Care: Some Crucial Distinctions." *Gerontologist* 28 (Supplement, June): 10–17.

Daniels, Norman. 1986. "Why Saying No to Patients in the United States Is So Hard." *New England Journal of Medicine* 314: 1380–83.

Dworkin, Gerald. 1978. "Moral Autonomy." In H. Tristram Engelhardt, Jr. and Daniel Callahan, eds., *Morals, Science and Sociality.* Hastings-on-Hudson, NY: Institute of Society, Ethics and the Life Sciences. pp. 156–171.

———. 1988. *The Theory and Practice of Autonomy*. Cambridge: Cambridge University Press.

Engelhardt, Jr., H. Tristram. 1982. "Bioethics in Pluralist Societies." *Perspectives in Biology and Medicine* 26: 64–78.

Faden, Ruth R., and Tom L. Beauchamp. 1986. *A History of Informed Consent*. New York and Oxford: Oxford University Press.

Feinberg, Joel. 1978. "The Interest in Liberty on the Scales." In A. Goldman and J. Kim, eds., *Values and Morals*. Dordrecht, Holland:

Gilman, Sander L. 1988. *Disease and Representation: Images of Illness from Madness to AIDS*. Ithaca, NY and London: Cornell University Press.

Glendon, Mary Ann. 1991. *Rights Talk: The Impoverishment of Political Discourse*. New York: MacMillan.

Hauerwas, Stanley J. 1981. *A Community of Character*. Notre Dame, IN: University of Notre Dame Press.

Haworth, Lawrence. 1986. *Autonomy: An Essay in Philosophical Psychology and Ethics*. New Haven, CT: Yale University Press.

Ladd, John. 1978. "Legalism and Medical Ethics." In John. W. Davis, Barry Hoffmaster, and Sarah Shorten, eds., *Contemporary Issues in Biomedical Ethics*. Clifton, NJ: Humana Press. pp. 1–35.

Larmore, Charles E. 1987. *Patterns of Moral Complexity*. Cambridge: Cambridge University Press.

Lidz, Charles W., Paul S. Appelbaum, and Alan Meisel. 1988. "Two Models of Implementing the Idea of Informed Consent." *Archives of Internal Medicine* 148: 1385–89.

MacIntyre, Alasdair. 1977. "Patients As Agents." In Stuart F. Spicker and H. Tristram Engelhardt, Jr., eds., *Philosophical Medical Ethics: Its Nature and Significance*. Dordrecht, Holland: D. Reidel Publishing Company. pp. 197–212.

———. 1981. *After Virtue: A Study in Moral Theory*. Notre Dame, IN: University of Notre Dame Press.

———. 1988. *Whose Justice? Which Rationality?* Notre Dame, IN: University of Notre Dame Press.

Mann, Thomas. 1967. *The Magic Mountain*. H. T. Lowe-Porter, trans. New York: McGraw.

Parsons, Talcott. 1958. "Definitions of Health and Illness in Light of American Values and Social Structure." In E. Gartley Jaco, ed., *Patients, Physicians, and Illness: Source Book in Behavioral Science and Medicine*. New York: Free Press. pp. 165–187.

Pellegrino, Edmund D., and Thomasma, David C. 1981. *A Philosophical Basis of Medical Practice*. New York and Oxford: Oxford University Press.

Perry, Michael J. 1988. *Morality, Politics and Law*. New York and Oxford: Oxford University Press.

Richards, David A. J. 1981. "Rights and Autonomy," *Ethics* 92 (1): 3–20.

Sandel, Michael. 1982. *Liberalism and the Limits of Justice.* New York: Cambridge University Press.

Schutz, Alfred. 1970. *Reflections on the Problem of Relevance.* Richard M. Zaner, ed. New Haven, CT: Yale University Press.

———. 1971a. *Collected Papers, I: The Problem of Social Reality.* Maurice Natanson, ed. The Hague: Martinus Nijhoff.

———. 1971b. *Collected Papers, II: Studies in Social Theory.* Arvid Brodersen, ed. The Hague: Martinus Nijhoff.

Thomasma, David C. 1984. "Competency, Dependency, and the Care of the Very Old." *Journal of the American Geriatrics Society* 32: 906–914.

Wellman, Carl. 1985. *A Theory of Rights: Persons Under Laws, Institutions, and Morals.* New York: Rowman and Allanheld.

Wolf, Stewart. 1961. "Disease as a Way of Life: Neural Integration in Systemic Pathology." *Perspectives in Biology and Medicine* 4 (Spring): 288–305.

Young, Robert B. 1986. *Personal Autonomy: Beyond Negative and Positive Liberty.* New York: St. Martin's Press.

Zaner, Richard M. 1981. *The Context of Self: A Phenomenological Inquiry Using Medicine as a Clue.* Athens, OH: Ohio University Press.

Zerubavel, Eviatar. 1979. *Patterns of Time in Hospital Life.* Chicago and London: University of Chicago Press.

———. 1981. *Hidden Rhythms: Schedules and Calendars in Social Life.* Chicago and London: University of Chicago Press.

8

DISABILITY AND THE PERSISTENCE OF THE "NORMAL"

JOHN W. DOUARD

We must stop talking and allow ourselves the luxury of *listening* to
the voices that stir the air. I will be told that I need to score the voices;
but the sounds of the city reverberate in the zone *between* noise and music.
That is my home.

"DISABILITY," "HANDICAP," "IMPAIRMENT": the meanings and references of these terms have changed over the last century because social change creates new categories and alters the extension of old categories. I shall discuss some of these changes below. Changes in the way we talk about people with physical or mental disabilities are examples of what Ian Hacking calls "making up people."[1]

One constant that links different disability classificatory schemes is the distinction between the normal and the abnormal (or subnormal). The distinction between people who are normal and people who are abnormal has been associated by some writers with premodern notions of an immutable human nature and a cosmology in which people were thought to have been arranged in a rigid hierarchical order.[2] I will not deny a premodern origin for the normal/abnormal distinction, but I believe a modern conception of what it is for a person to be normal emerged in Europe and the United States during the last half of the nineteenth century.

In this essay I shall examine two competing models of disability: the functional limitations model and the minority group model. I shall argue that both models depend, in very different ways, on a common cognitive style which classifies people in terms of their relationship to a social norm. That cognitive style emerged in the nineteenth century in conjunction with an obsession for measuring deviance. As Michel Foucault writes:

... the marks that once indicated status, privilege, affiliation were increasingly replaced ... by a whole range of degrees of normality indicating membership of a homogeneous social body. ... In a sense, the power of normalization imposes homogeneity; but it individualizes by making it possible to measure gaps, to determine levels, to fix specialties, and to render the differences useful by fitting them one to another. It is easy to understand how the power of the norm functions within a system of formal equality, since within a homogeneity that is the rule, the norm introduces, as a useful imperative and as a result of measurement, all the shading of individual differences.[3]

The simultaneous use of "normal" as a result of measurement and as a social imperative introduces a crucial ambiguity into the distinction between the normal and the abnormal. This distinction, I believe, shapes both models.

I shall begin with an analysis of the notion of disease as a deviation from normal functional organization. My analysis will be in part historical, since I believe this conception of disease emerged at a time in which virtually every form of deviance, including disability, became medicalized.

Next, I shall examine the functional limitations and the minority group models of disability. I shall argue that the cognitive style of both models presupposes the evaluative and descriptive senses of "normal." This should come as a surprise to proponents of both models. What is really at issue *is the fundamentally coercive nature of social strategies for creating and sustaining a disciplined work force.* Neither model of disability adequately addresses these strategies.

Finally, I shall argue that an examination of disability policy reveals an unjustifiable reliance on public policy to solve the dilemma created when people who are very different from one another try to prohibit differences. I begin with a historical sketch of the role of the concept of normality in constructing disability policy.

The Normal and the Abnormal

Ian Hacking has pointed out that around 1820 an "avalanche of numbers" began that was obsessed with the statistics of deviance.[4] More generally, in the nineteenth century, a variety of disciplines set about devising techniques for measuring deviations from normal states or conditions. Adolphe Quételet's statistical notion of the "average man" transformed description of statistical regularities into laws of human nature and society, and by the end of the century Francis Galton had introduced the statistical and eugenic concept of "regression to the mean" into the vocabulary of social science. In medicine, the measurement of deviations from normal functional organization became the cornerstone of a nonvitalist pathology. If, in contrast to a hypothetical vital force, life is nothing but the result of external or internal physical stimulation, then one should be able to devise an experimental method for measuring a normal range of physiological functioning. Deviation from that normal range is the result of an excess or deficiency of excitation. Thus, according to Broussais, a physiological (and therefore, in his view, scientific) pathology consists in discovering how "this excitation can deviate from the normal state and constitute an abnormal or diseased state."[5] This is a putatively value-neutral conception of pathology.

Prior to the nineteenth century, disease had been thought to have its own unique essence, qualitatively distinct from, and always threatening, health. By 1850, health and disease were ranged along a continuum. Life and death were no longer tragically opposed forces, with death always beyond the reach of reason, but were part of the same process and open to scientific investigation. From that moment to the present, sickness was no longer to be considered an enchanted state,[6] but something that must be brought under the control of scientific experts.

The germ theory of disease brought medical expertise and political order together. Deborah Stone suggests that by the end of the nineteenth century, the germ theory of disease supplanted virtually all other theories in Europe and America as explanation of diseases, including functional impairments.[7] Her reason for stressing this point is that physicians came to be considered as having special expertise in diagnosing and measuring deviations from physiological norms, largely because of the germ theory. But even before the germ theory, the conception of pathology pioneered by Bichat and refined by Bernard had already initiated modern scientific medicine. Furthermore, prior to the germ theory physiological pathology had placed disease and physical impairment beyond the control of the sick person. A more important result of the germ theory, in connection with disability, is that it placed the responsibility on the police power of the state to implement public health measures. A link was forged between medical theory and politics that required statistical techniques for measuring minute differences between people, and for placing them in disease categories.[8]

The influence of these developments in medicine shaped the concept of disability. A disability came to be understood as a dysfunctional, and therefore an abnormal, physical or psychological condition. Kenneth Hamilton's distinction, drawn in 1950, between "disability" and "handicap" came after a century of influential medical thinking about disability:

A disability is a condition of impairment, physical or mental, having an objective aspect that can usually be described by a physician. It is a medical thing. A handicap is the cumulative result of the obstacles which disability interposes between the individual and his maximum functional level. . . . It is an individual thing.[9]

In short, a disability is the medical condition the physician can diagnose and treat; a handicap is the set of obstacles disabled persons must confront. Hamilton clearly believes that the "maximum functional level" of a person is the level at which a typical, or average, person can perform. The emphasis on "objective" conditions and "maximum functional levels" represents an effort to identify a value-neutral core of the disability category.

Beginning in the nineteenth century, medicine successfully claimed the authority to diagnose, treat, and measure deviance. That authority was socially constructed, as was the medical realism on which the authority was largely based. What Arnold Davidson has said of perversion can also be said of many conditions, including disability:

Perversion was not a disease that lurked about in nature, waiting for a psychiatrist [or physiologist] with especially acute powers of observation to discover it hiding everywhere. It was a disease created by a new functional understanding of disease.[10]

Auguste Comte transferred the physiologists' conception of the "normal state" to the state itself:

Until Broussais, the pathological state obeyed laws completely different from those governing the normal state. . . . Broussais established that the phenomena of disease are of essentially the same kind as those of health, from which they differed only in intensity. The collective organism, because of its greater degree of complexity, is liable to problems more serious, varied, and frequent than those of the individual organism. I do not hesitate to state that Broussais's principle must be extended to this point and I have often applied it to confirm or perfect sociological laws.[11]

Now, the descriptive/normative ambiguity of "normal" lurks in the physiologists' conception of normal functioning as an ideal of perfection as well as an objective description of a state of affairs.[12] In Comte, the same ambiguity is transferred to the state along with the medical analogy: deviation from the positive laws of normal social functioning are problems that the sociologist can study. Social problems are the sociologist's laboratory, just as pathological conditions of an organism are the physiologist's laboratory. The obvious implication is that the normal state of society can be described as functional integrity, and that functional integrity is the mark of a good, or healthy, society.

In light of the valorization of the normal state, certain social problems of long standing have special significance as markers of major social and cultural upheavals. One such problem is vagrancy: how ought institutions to deal with the fact that some people either cannot, or will not, work. The category of disability is connected historically with legal categories created during the transition from a feudal mode of production in Europe to a commercial mode of production. This transition involved, among other things, an increase in social and geographical mobility; a change from largely task-oriented, small-scale production to the employed labor of large-scale machine-driven industry; a complex division of labor; and the construction of an objective, finely calibrated measure of time (embodied in the clock) in an effort to create regular labor rhythms. Socially, the transition was characterized, in part, by a move away from a social hierarchy based on traditional ties to land and lord, to a hierarchy based on one's place in the employed labor force. This was the social and economic context in which Europe's nation-states emerged. The social and personal dislocations created by the transformations of modernity forced the new political orders to codify policies for the regulation of vagrancy.[13]

In this transition, two distinctions emerged that were to have important consequences for the category of disability: 1) work was separated spatially and temporally from the rest of life; and 2) subjective time was subordinated to the objective time required by large-scale employment.[14] These distinctions were preconditions of two developments in the nineteenth-century conceptualization of work. First, wage labor came to be the dominant normative force in structuring a person's life. A normal life came to be seen as one that is structured by a highly specific time discipline with employed labor at its center. Work is the center both of a day in a person's life and of the course of an entire life. Second, the time spent *not* working in a normal life is both trivialized and problematized. It is trivialized because it does not contribute to the worker's productivity. It is problematized because it can detract from productivity. Furthermore, socially valued work was fragmented into highly differentiated tasks performed under the surveillance of an employer. The commodification of work, space, and time as a *moral* order is reflected in the work of "industrial engineers" in the twentieth century. Thus, Kerr and Siegel write that structuring a labor force

involves the setting of rules on times to work and not work, on method and amount of pay, on movement into and out of work and from one position to another. It involves rules pertaining to the maintenance of continuity in the work process ... the attempted minimization of individual or organized revolt, the provision of view of the world, of ideological orientations, of beliefs. ... [15]

This rationalized vision of social life, which took shape in the nineteenth century, cannot easily incorporate a refusal to work according to plan (a form of "individual revolt") or an inability to work. The modern welfare state, which began more than a century ago in Europe, can be viewed as an effort to discipline employment outliers. But to maximize the public good, *categories* of outliers that marked important distinctions needed to be devised. Some people were unemployed because they were vagrants or malingerers, some because they were displaced by changes in the job market, and some because they were disabled, sick, or old. According to Stone, categories of theoretically nonstigmatizing work exemption were created as "a response to a long-standing policy dilemma: how to reconcile the distributive principles of work and need without undermining the productive side of the economy."[16]

In the nineteenth century, then, new categories were created, as a result of social change, that created "new ways for people to be." One can think of the welfare state as an elaborate political intervention, analogous to a medical intervention, to align unemployment and employment patterns, i.e., to normalize the abnormal. Thus, not only were space, time, and labor commodified, producing a new conception of what it is to be normal, but disability itself was commodified. The disability category was, and is, part of a welfare-state capitalist system of production and distribution. One result of the creation of disability categories was the creation of new medical specialties, because these categories rely heavily on the concept of physical and mental impairment, as diagnosed by morally neutral medical experts.

In the next two sections of this essay, I shall examine two current competing models of disability against the background of the foregoing historical sketch of the social construction of disability. Both models, I argue, are shaped by that history. One model is not as politically neutral as it claims to be. The other model is not as politically radical as it claims to be.

Disabled Persons or Disabled Societies?

I have pointed out that historically disability policy has been linked, on the one hand, to the concept of a "normal" range of employment opportunities and, on the other hand, to the concept of a "normal" range of physiological or psychological functional capacities. Medical diagnosis of total functional impairment is a putatively "objective" or value-neutral test of legitimate, nonstigmatized work exemption. Evidence that one suffers from prolonged incapacity, despite the likelihood of stigma in certain areas of social life, places one in a category that is relatively free from pressures to rejoin the labor force. Unlike public assistance or temporary illness, prolonged incapacity caused by total functional impairment can therefore be viewed as nonstigmatizing in the sphere of work. As Haber and Smith put it, "labeling role failure as disability reduces critical evaluation by neutralizing conventional norms and by offering adaptive alternatives."[17] The authors also point out that administrative requirements of "simplicity, standardization, and reliability for routinized decision-making" lead to a definition of disability based at least in part on attributes such as functional impairment rather than on limitations of social roles. The attribution of functional impairments to the disabled is the heart of the functional limitations model of disability.

The Functional Limitations Model (FLMD)

As I noted above, Kenneth Hamilton drew a distinction between "impairment" or "disability" and the obstacles that constitute "handicap." The functional limitations model of disability requires some such distinction. But Hamilton attributes both the impairment and the obstacles to the disabled person. Since then, much has been written about the social construction of disability, and current versions of the FLMD take this work into account.

It is a mistake, I believe, to claim that the functional limitations model is committed to the view that *disabilities* are essential attributes of certain individuals.[18] The version of the FLMD I shall examine here attributes functional limitations, but not disabilities, to individuals. Functional limitations are, in this version, deviations from species-typical functioning or from statistical norms. In either case, functional limitations are presumed to be real, theory-independent properties that define a category of persons. Thus, Saad Nagi constructs a disability trajectory with the following nodes:

1) active pathology, i.e., interruption of normal physiological processes;

2) impairment, i.e., loss or abnormality of function at the level of organ systems;

3) functional limitations; i.e., manifestations of impairment at the level of the organism as a whole;

4) disability, i.e., inability or limitation in performing socially defined roles and tasks expected of an individual within a socio-cultural environment and physical environment.[19]

It is important to understand that Nagi's distinctions are not simply academic exercises. They have important policy implications. In the first place, the reference to "socially defined roles" in clause 4 considerably generalizes from the earlier focus on the single social role of work to so-called "activities of daily living." To the extent that activities of daily living fall within the scope of public institutions, such as antidiscrimination laws, state interventions may be justified to structure the environment in such a way as to ensure access by disabled persons. Thus the Americans With Disabilities Act (ADA) is intended to remove or change features of the human environment that are likely to prevent people with disabilities from engaging in those activities to which all citizens have a right. Nagi's model can be construed as providing scientific warrant for such policies.

Also, people with disabilities may be eligible for benefits under either Social Security Disability Insurance or Supplemental Security Income. SSDI and SSI benefits are based on somewhat different eligibility criteria. Thus, SSDI may provide benefits to persons who become impaired after a period of employment; SSI benefits may cover persons who are impaired from birth. As Lance Liebman points out, the former is a straightforward entitlement based on the working individual's contribution made to the public good. In a sense, the "public" acts as insurers, and work is a kind of premium payment. SSI, however, is essentially a welfare privilege, qualified by the assumption that persons disabled at birth are not to blame for their condition. The social norm for assessing claims under both policies is income-producing work.[20]

Among the SSI and the SSDI eligibility requirements is the condition that the impairment or functional limitation be medically determinable and total. The ADA marks off the category it covers more broadly: it defines a disability "with respect to an individual" as "a physical or mental impairment that substantially limits one or more of the major life activities of such an individual; a record of such an impairment; or being regarded as having such an impairment."[21] The ADA does not explicitly define "impairment," but it is conceptually and historically tied to the Rehabilitation Act of 1973, which does define "impairment" as a medically diagnosable condition.

Hence, Nagi's version of the FLMD, the SSI, the SSDI, and the ADA all define "disability" in terms of a medically diagnosable impairment or functional limitation, which is presumed to be a quality of individuals that is independent of their relation to social structure. Put another way, the presumption is that normal functioning is a property of individuals in virtue of which they are biologically normal members of a species. Notice, however, that the judgment that someone falls within a normal range of species-typical functioning is ambiguous: it simultaneously *describes* and *evaluates* them.

Thus, Nagi refers to normal performance levels as "optimal," and in so doing he plays on the ambiguity of "normal" by covertly presupposing that it is *desirable* to function normally. On the one hand, Nagi claims to be modeling, on the basis of empirical data, the process of becoming disabled. This is a descriptive claim. On the other hand, he clearly takes a normative stance toward the normal: to be normal is to be "all right."[22] Like Comte, proponents of the functional limitations model of disability let the word "normal" do two jobs: presenting a true description of a state of affairs, and evaluating it morally. In effect, they make two power moves. The first move is the assertion that they (i.e., the experts) have the authority to determine the truth. Experts can model reality. The second move is to convey, usually implicitly, that they also have the authority to assess the desirability of levels of performance. The important point is that *both moves are made simultaneously*, within the same "discursive practice."[23]

The FLMD is coercive in the same way that the modern factory is coercive. Both are rationalized as empirically grounded representations, of disabilities and of efficient production respectively, and therefore as in some sense natural. *When people with disabilities, the professionals who care for them, and the rest of the community* give assent to the knowledge produced by experts, we are all "vehicles of power." Constraint becomes self-constraint; coercion becomes discipline.[24]

The FLMD eliminates all qualitative differences in favor of quantitative differences. Consider someone who has permanently lost the use of a limb. In one sense she is quite different from me: I can use all my limbs. From the point of view of the FLMD, however, the only difference between us is that she cannot perform as many social roles and tasks as I can. We are not radically different. There is no place in the model for a phenomenology of difference; that is, there is no way to represent our very different *experiences of living*. The FLMD is an "objective" model, and cannot capture the key feature of human experience: subjectivity or point of view. To say that someone is a subject is to say there is *something it is like to be* that person.[25]

The FLMD doesn't capture what it is like to be a particular person with a particular disability because it is an abstraction. The model, like all models, abstracts from the particulars of the lived experiences of people with disabilities. It is, of course, a statistical view, and it is the outcome of concrete social practices engaged in by the experts. Hence, it is *not* what it purports to be.

These points constitute a critique of the FLMD: the fundamental problem with the model is that it presupposes that social scientists and other experts have the authority to draw a distinction between the normal and the abnormal. Like all models, it is an abstraction that homogenizes the myriad experiences of living with a disability in order to measure minute, objective deviations from social norms of appearance and ability. Those norms are embodied in institutions, among which are the social and medical sciences themselves.

In a recent article, neurologist Oliver Sacks captures the difficulty one runs up against when disabilities are medicalized as quantitative deviations from norms. He describes a young man, Gregg, who is "stuck" in the 1960s: the world's last hippie. Gregg was discovered in 1975 to have a benign but massive brain tumor. The tumor caused a number of specific neurological "deficits," but also a more global disturbance of the self associated with damage to the frontal lobes. Gregg's parents, who had not seen him for four years while the tumor had gone untreated, thought that "he was changed beyond recognition, had been 'dispossessed,' in his father's words." Sacks speaks of "neurological deficits" unreflexively until he writes:

> Though, as a neurologist, I had to speak of his "syndrome," his "deficits," I did not feel this was adequate to describe Gregg. I felt, one felt, he had become another "kind" of person; that though his functional lobe damage had taken away his identity in a way, yet it had also given him a sort of identity or personality, albeit of an odd and perhaps primitive sort.[26]

When Sacks stepped out of his role as a neurologist, he no longer felt compelled to see Gregg as simply deviating from a normal or species-typical range of functional organization. Gregg can be spoken of as having a certain sort of identity typical of people with frontal lobe damage. Relative to *that* class, Gregg is "normal."

None of this is to say, of course, that Gregg's condition is not tragic. He is unable to engage in performances most of us take for granted, largely because he has little or no capacity to move information from short-term to long-term memory. But it is noteworthy that he has a personality, in Sacks's view: in particular, Gregg responds with an unusual depth (for him) to music, for which he has a talent. Had Sacks confined himself to assessing Gregg's neurological deficits, rather than noticing and responding to contexts in which Gregg's personality emerges, there is a sense in which he would never have come to know Gregg at all.

The belief that impairments and the functional limitations caused by impairments are occurrent, monadic properties of individuals in virtue of which they deviate from species-typical functioning is illusory. People are impaired, as well as disabled, relative to a population of people who are judged to be normal. However, the standards of normal functioning are constructed from the point of view of people who satisfy the standards. Indeed, those standards are negotiated, and not discovered or diagnosed. There is no reason *in principle* why physiological and psychological capacities that are now taken to fall outside the normal range should not be taken as normal, had these standards been negotiated differently. In short, *I suggest that reality is negotiated socially,* including what we call impairments. Irving Zola, at the end of *Missing Pieces,* his narrative of disability, writes:

> Where once social rhetoric made reference to good and evil, legal and illicit, now it refers to "healthy" and "sick." We are experiencing a medicalization of society and with it the growth of medicine as an institution and instrument of social control.[27]

Now, I do not believe this is a *morally* objectionable state of affairs. From what vantage point could I justify such a judgment? Indeed, given the power of the institutions of science and medicine in our culture, I suspect it is inevitable. That is an empirical claim it would take me too far afield to argue here. Instead, I would like to turn my attention to another feature of the functional limitations model of disability: it assumes, usually implicitly, that there is a normal range of social roles.

This assumption is implicit in Nagi's definition of disability. Recall that he defines disability as "an inability or limitation in performing socially defined roles." Disability is still attributed *to an individual* relative to social role expectations that are constructed by institutions designed to accommodate people without those limitations. One might ask, however, why Nagi doesn't define disability as a property of the role expectations themselves. Admittedly, that would sound odd, but as a philosopher I am entitled to ask odd questions. There is no reason *in principle* that I can think of why we do not call social role expectations disabled relative to the full range of human capacities, unless we believe that those role expectations are *normal.*

That we do indeed believe role expectations to be normal, both descriptively and evaluatively, is suggested by the fact that we sometimes change our expectations when they are challenged as abnormal relative to some people's capacities. Thus, role expectations of women started to change when enough women charged that those expectations did not match their capacities. The disability rights movement is also making the point that there is nothing normal, in a purely descriptive sense, about role expectations. Thus, social norms are changing, not simply because society is disabling, but because it is disabled: it is unable to adapt to some people's capacities.

There are political reasons why modern societies make the distinctions between normal and deviant functioning and normal and deviant role performance. The main reason, judging from the social history I sketched earlier, is that we want policies that can identify malingerers, discourage dependence, and meet needs. Such policies are strategies of social control that came to dominate Western societies to address problems raised by the creation of a labor market and a capitalist mode of production.

Institutions are not infinitely plastic, but they can change. When they do, norms, perceptions, and thought change as well. Here, then, is another problem with the FLMD, in addition to its essentialist conception of functional limitations: it seems to hold institutions stable, and focuses on altering the capacities of people who fall short of the norms. Indeed, the claim of the FLMD to value-neutrality *entails* that it cannot evaluate institutions and their ends. This is not so for the minority group model of disability. To see why, I need to spell out the minority group model in somewhat more detail. Unfortunately, it also seems to rely on the disability category to the extent that it identifies a distinct minority group.[28]

The Minority Group Model (MGMD)

The MGMD makes use of a relatively new moral language. Minority group models claim, among other things, that groups, as well as (and, occasionally, instead of) individuals, are subjects of rights. Later I shall discuss several problems with this claim. The MGMD deserves careful attention, however, because of its strengths: first, it is situated in the experience of living with a disability; second, it challenges the dominant culture to justify its power to make decisions for the disabled; third, it is the foundation for an effective political strategy.

The proponents of the MGMD claim the model is situated in the experience of living with a disability, and "encompasses ethical values that cannot be totally ignored by health professionals and others in vocations that involve extensive work with disabled clients."[29] Perhaps the most important of these values is expressed in the belief that life with a disability can be rewarding, creative, dignified, and, all in all, worth living. That this is often *not* the case is the result of a social environment that is itself disabling for people with physical and mental limitations, in part because society labels such limitations as disabilities. As Harlan

Hahn puts it: "The 'minority group' paradigm is based on a socio-political defini-tion of disability as a product of the interaction between the individual and the environment." [30]

The result of labeling is discrimination against a distinct minority group—people with disabilities—on the basis of personal characteristics that ought to be morally and politically irrelevant. The principle of fair equality of opportunity in the broadest sense is abrogated in the case of people with disabilities. The MGMD is incorporated in the Americans With Disabilities Act:

> (7) individuals with disabilities are a discrete and insular minority who have been faced with restrictions and limitations, subjected to a history of purposeful un-equal treatment, and relegated to a position of political powerlessness in our so-ciety . . .

> (8) the Nation's proper goals regarding individuals with disabilities are to assure equality of opportunity, full participation, independent living, and economic self-sufficiency for such individuals. [31]

The MGMD has important consequences for bioethics and social policy. The received view of the ethics of medical decision-making, for example, emphasizes patient autonomy as the basis for a right to "voluntary, informed choice." But, according to Arthur Caplan et al., "The capacity for free, voluntary choices may have to be facilitated in patients since it may be unrealistic to expect such capaci-ties to be present in those who have suffered grievous and irreversible impair-ments." [32] Who is to "facilitate" patient autonomy in these cases, according to Cap-lan? The rehabilitation specialists, whose "clinical experience with patients who suffered severe disability, injury, or disease makes them skeptical about the ability patients possess to make informed, deliberate, and reasoned choices concerning risks and benefits of treatment." [33] The authors of this report clearly presuppose the functional limitations model of disability. How would decision making about choices faced by people with disabilities be structured if one presupposed the mi-nority group model?

The decision-making process would be distributed differently, for one thing. The MGMD would place decisions in the hands of people with disabilities. It would replace control over those decisions by professional experts with control by people with disabilities and their communities. Indeed, the MGMD could en-courage a different perspective on technical expertise: people with disabilities who have learned to cope with a relatively unfriendly social world can provide expert advice to the newly disabled, ethics committees, physicians, rehabilitation counselors, genetic counselors, and other professionals about a wide range of ethical and social problems. Most importantly, the nature of disability would be reconceptualized to remove the stigma attached to disability, and to shift the goal of rehabilitation away from accommodation and acceptance to the development of creative new ways of living well with impairments.

The MGMD also has enormous implications for social policy. Consider the current interest, among health administrators, physicians, and rehabilitation professionals, in health outcomes assessment. The interest has been fostered in part by skepticism about the value of physician discretion and by economic pressure to reduce health care costs. Outcomes assessment and formal models of medical decision making are considered by many health professionals to be the best way to begin standardizing treatment choices. The goal is to construct "practice policies" based on statistical analysis of treatment outcomes.[34] The strategies for constructing practice policies, however, cannot in principle include the perspective of patients themselves. If a similar approach to disability rehabilitation is pursued, the functional limitations model is likely to be the model of disability considered most appropriate. Standardized rehabilitation practices may be developed by experts, and their implementation may be determined by experts and administrators. The sorts of concerns Caplan et al. articulate will shape the formulation of rehabilitation practice policies. According to critics of the FLMD, these concerns are a consequence of the normalizing imperative of the model. The minority group model would eliminate the normalizing imperative itself, and thus would reduce the role of specialized rehabilitation expertise in decision making. (It may also, of course, entail rejecting the initial move toward standardizing practice policies.)

Notice that the minority group model is not, on the face of it, incompatible with the functional limitations model. Descriptively, to say that a person has functional limitations is to say she/he does not fall within a normal range of functional capacities. As we have seen, Nagi makes the descriptive claim that disabilities are the result of interaction between functional limitations and social structure. Nothing prohibits proponents of the FLMD from holding that people with disabilities constitute a minority group that has been the focus of social discrimination. Indeed, much of Hahn's own vision of the advantages of the MGMD can also be held by proponents of the FLMD: the latter can believe just as fervently as the former that people with functional limitations can flourish.

One important difference between the models, however, is that proponents of MGMD tend to view the FLMD as itself a site of the power of experts to label people as disabled, with the result that persons so labeled are disempowered. The strength of the MGMD lies in its refusal to accept uncritically the claim made on behalf of the FLMD that expert judgment is value-neutral. Functional limitations only serve as a test of disability, according to the MGMD, when social roles themselves are held immune from criticism. The power embedded in social relations is then left unchallenged by medical and disability rehabilitation experts. By laying bare the role of power in defining disability, the MGMD opens the way for articulation of a social vision that holds all forms of social power to be contestable.

The MGMD, however, must confront a serious conceptual and practical difficulty. We have gotten used to the idea that rights can sensibly be claimed by an oppressed minority group, and even though a collectivist approach to rights is often contested, it has received considerable jurisprudential support over the last fifteen years. Now, the legal categories of group identity are intended to "carve the universe at a natural joint," which in this context means a natural *social* joint.[35] But to what social group do all people with disabilities belong? A social group is defined, in part, by a common culture; and members of a legally designated disadvantaged group belong to a common subculture. A common subculture can provide its members with sources of values and goals that are distinct from, and sometimes opposed to, dominant values and goals. Without a common subculture, anything that accentuates differences in kind rather than differences in degree can seem to increase vulnerability rather than pride. People with disabilities, however, do not share a common subculture.

I suspect that one very important reason for this problem is precisely that, unlike people of color and women, people with disabilities have for over a century been identified as quantitatively (but not qualitatively) deviating from the normal. I have argued that the medicalization of disability and the centrality of work in modern societies are largely responsible for this vision of disability. The MGMD must counter a deeply entrenched perception, which is that the disabled do not form a distinct cultural group.

Furthermore, there is a strong presumption in the United States that, even if cultural identity ought not be melted down, social opportunities ought to be available on the basis of merit. When minority groups challenge meritocratic principles, and claim collective rights, they run the danger of being accused of subordinating individual differences to group identity. The identity politics of the MGMD raises the spector of essentialism: in virtue of what objective properties can people with disabilities claim membership in a distinct minority group? If the properties are the functional limitations of the socially constructed category adopted by the FLMD, then the models are not clearly distinct from one another.

If the MGMD rejects functional limitations as the metaphysical basis of its identification of a minority group, it requires some other criteria of membership.

Even if the MGMD could provide nonessentialist criteria of membership, there are problems with identity politics itself. One's personal identity is surely shaped to a great extent by one's group identity, but not entirely. If one's identification with a single group is too tight, one's ability to flourish can be stifled. The tradition of individual rights derives much of its appeal from the protection it affords *individuals* from complete submersion in *any* group. There is a risk that the MGMD can lead to such an effacement of individual differences.

Furthermore, minority group models tend to subordinate all cultural and social differences to a single characteristic that members of groups share. In modern, pluralist societies, individuality is often highly valued; but in addition, each of us belongs to several groups with which we more or less identify, and which shape our conceptions of the good life. Minority group models, to the extent that they minimize the importance of such multiple allegiances, can suppress the very real tensions some of their members may feel about isolating *one*, usually stigmatizing, characteristic as representing them. Whether or not essentialism is good metaphysics, it can create a kind of psychological dissonance when it shapes social taxonomy.

I have argued that the identity politics of the MGMD can promote local homogeneity within the minority group the dominant culture labels as disabled. I do not deny the political exigencies of organizing a disability rights movement. Nor do I deny the importance of using that movement to ensure fair equality of opportunity. Policies such as the ADA, however much they may leave untouched the ubiquitous commodification of modern life, can be used to serve the interests of the disabled, just as the civil rights laws can be used to serve the interests of other oppressed groups.

Furthermore, disability rights advocates have demonstrated a tradition of oppression that has done far more to inhibit individual flourishing than has identification with a minority group. The MGMD shows that adaptation to the social norms of the white, middle-class, male majority is as unreasonable an expectation for the disabled as it is for members of other minority groups. That will require showing that the perception of disability as mere quantitative deviation from the normal state is mistaken. Hahn makes the point clearly:

> . . . limitations labelled as disabilities have been viewed . . . as pathological conditions to be eradicated or remedied to the maximum extent possible. Rather

these limitations could be viewed simply as additional manifestations of the diversity of human attributes which may become a source of prejudice in a culture that imposes a high degree of conformity on the characteristics of its members.[36]

The Politics of Difference

The political vision of modernity gains much of its plausibility from its close association with modern science.[37] Scientists use a common method for arriving at theoretical agreement, and its success is measured by the remarkable degree to which science can control natural phenomena and render experience intelligible to any rational agent. If political institutions can use analogous methods for exercising social control, freedom and order may both be realized. The key idea linking modern science and modern politics is that we can arrive at least at the simulacrum of truth in politics if we construct policies that can control and rationalize social relations.

It is this link between science and politics that has seemed to lend weight to modern notions of normalcy. When society shifted from status to contract, a new center of social order was required to replace the earlier hierarchical arrangement based on one's relationship to king and land. Scientists seemed to have discovered that there is a lawful natural order that can be experimentally distorted and then measured.

In their historical analysis of the dispute between Thomas Hobbes and Robert Boyle over the relationship that ought to obtain between science and the polity, Steven Shapin and Simon Schaffer write: "Scientific activity, the scientist's role, and the scientific community have always been dependent: they exist, are valued, and [are] supported insofar as the state or its various agencies see point in them."[38]

This dependency continued into the nineteenth century, when current disability policies originated in the United States. I have argued that central to this dependency was an analogy between the human body and the social body. Disease seems to provide an experimental field for discovering how the *body's* natural order is distorted by outside forces. Perhaps the *social* body has a natural order that is distorted by social forces: just as experiments and disease cause deviations from a natural order, so social forces cause deviations from a social order. The center of the modern social order is work, since work is just the expenditure necessary to survive and flourish. Within this framework, social roles can be defined that regiment human behavior in order to maximize productivity and consumption. The mirror image of this functional approach to controlling the social body is a functional approach to controlling the sick or disabled body.

Unlike technical errors in science or criminal behavior in the polity, however, disability and chronic illness seem not to be under complete human control. They are deviations from both the natural order and the social order for which no individual can be held responsible, and which neither science nor politics can eliminate. Disability is a constant reminder that the fantasy of complete control *cannot* be realized.

The fantasy of control, however, articulates with the belief that either scientific progress or well-designed social arrangements (or perhaps both) can resolve what Martha Minow calls "the dilemma of difference."[39] According to Minow, there are two dominant strategies for preventing the stigmatization of people who are different, both of which are self-defeating. One strategy is to integrate those who are different with the dominant culture by "erasing" their differences. This strategy recommends the development of scientific and therapeutic techniques for reducing or eliminating the respects in which people with disabilities deviate from biological norms. This is, roughly, the strategy at the heart of the functional limitations model of disability.

The other strategy is to define a class of people who are different, and to modify or eliminate the social structures that handicap them. This strategy recommends disability policies that alter social structure, such as the Americans With Disabilities Act. This is, roughly, the strategy at the heart of the minority group model of disability.

Now, both of these strategies may well alleviate some of the problems of living of some people with disabilities. On the one hand, technological innovation has resulted in prosthetic devices that enable the disabled, and therapeutic innovation has reduced the disabling character of physical or mental disabilities. On the other hand, policies such as the ADA are likely to remove at least some of the disabling features of the social environment that simply are not designed to accommodate people with disabilities.

Nonetheless, both strategies help sustain stigmatization of the disabled. Efforts to integrate people with disabilities into the dominant culture can create a class of second-class citizens, since differences often cannot be erased. If the social environment remains unchanged, people with disabilities that cannot be eliminated continue to suffer discrimination. Indeed, discrimination may well be intensified, since the social conditions of self-respect remain linked to social and biological norms.

Both the FLMD and the MGMD look to public policy for solutions to the dilemmas created by ineliminable differences among people. Public policies are required to secure protection of vulnerable citizens from oppressive social structures, to protect everyone from violence, and to secure the "health of the Republic." I suggest, however, that public policy, in trying to accomplish these goals, can also institutionalize conformity and discipline.

On the one hand, efforts to alter social structures in response to the attribution of special rights to the disabled as members of a distinct minority group institutionalize the social process of labeling. Such policies emphasize a single defining feature of the group—disability—at the expense of intragroup diversity and individuality. On the other hand, efforts to secure health by defining a normal body statistically can also institutionalize stigma and discrimination of those who do not "qualify" as normal. People with disabilities are assigned the task of "improving" their bodies prosthetically if they wish to be integrated into the social order. Such policies render the oppressive features of the status quo invisible.

The dilemma of difference cannot be resolved unless we recognize the link between socially constructed norms and the political culture of modernity. If uncontrollable deviations from the normal are inevitable, and if modern life is largely oriented toward eliminating such deviations, the result is what Friedrich Nietzsche called *ressentiment. Ressentiment* is the obsessive refusal to acknowledge disorder as a permanent condition of humankind, a condition that cannot be eliminated by either love or domination. When we insist that every human problem can be solved, and normalcy restored, failure is inevitable. The result is usually fear, anger, or the pretense that the differences do not exist or do not matter. As William Connolly puts it:

> The modern normal, responsible individual can redirect resentment against the human condition into the self, first, by treating the rational, self-interested, free, and principled individual as morally responsible for willful deviations from normal identity and, second, by treating that in itself and other selves which falls below the threshold of responsibility as a natural defect in need of conquest or conversion, punishment or love.[40]

The result is a politics that tries to eliminate deviations from the normal, rather than a politics that promotes the association of persons who are different from one another.

What Connolly articulates in this passage is a deep conflict of values that is rarely addressed in modern political discourse: on the one hand, individuals are to be held responsible for their actions, and, on the other hand, individuals ought not to be held responsible if their actions deviate too far from standards of normality. From this perspective, neither attributions of responsibility nor standards of normality are to be challenged, because they help constitute the values that frame political discourse itself.

I have argued here that these assumptions of modern political discourse, and the political order that sustains that discourse, can be challenged by a critical examination of the two dominant models of disability. I have argued, further, that unless we examine critically the limits of public policy to solve our problems of living together, exemplified by disability policies, we may not notice the ways such policies enforce and sustain conformity and discipline.

NOTES

1. I. Hacking, "Making Up People," in *Reconstructing Individualism*, ed. T. C. Heller, M. Sosna, and D. E. Wellbery (Stanford: Stanford University Press, 1986), pp. 222–236.

2. M. Minow, *Making All the Difference* (Ithaca: Cornell University Press, 1990), pp. 105–107.

3. M. Foucault, *Discipline and Punish* (New York: Random House, 1979), p. 184.

4. I. Hacking, *The Taming of Chance* (Cambridge: Cambridge University Press, 1986), pp. 115–124.

5. Quoted in G. Canguilhem, *The Normal and the Pathological* (Cambridge, Mass.: The MIT Press, 1989), p. 54.

6. "The fate of our times is characterized by rationalization and intellectualization and, above all, by the 'disenchantment of the world.' Precisely the ultimate and most sublime values have retreated from public life either into the transcendental realm of mystic life or into the brotherliness of direct and personal human relations." M. Weber, "Science as a Vocation," in *From Max Weber*, ed. H. H. Gerth and C. W. Mills (Oxford: Oxford University Press, 1946), p. 155.

7. D. Stone, *The Disabled Society* (Philadelphia: Temple University Press, 1984), pp. 90–117.

8. Hacking, "Making Up People," p. 222.

9. K. Hamilton, *Counseling the Handicapped* (New York: The Ronald Press Company, 1950), p. 17.

10. Quoted in Hacking, "Making Up People," p. 222.

11. Quoted in G. Canguilhem, *The Normal and the Pathological*, p. 49.

12. Canguilhem, *The Normal and the Pathological*, pp. 238–239.

13. E. P. Thompson, "Time, Work Discipline, and Industrial Capitalism," *Past and Present* 38(Dec. 1967): 56–97.

14. Ibid., pp. 90–94.

15. C. Kerr and A. Siegel, "The Structuring of the Labor Force in Industrial Society: New Dimensions and New Questions," *Industrial and Labor Relations Review* 2(1955): 163.

16. Stone, *The Disabled Society*, p. 51.

17. L. D. Haber and R. T. Smith, "Disability and Deviance: Normative Adaptations of Role Behavior," *American Sociological Review* 36(February 1971): 94.

18. There is a growing critical literature on essentialism in scientific explanations, which I think is relevent to medical explanations of disabilities in terms of functional limitations. It is beyond the scope of this paper to discuss this literature in detail, but a good recent discussion of biological essentialism, and references to key texts in philosophy of science on the subject, can be found in J. Dupre, *The Disorder of Things: Metaphysical Foundations of the Disunity of Science* (Cambridge, Mass.: Harvard University Press, 1993), pp. 60–84.

19. S. Z. Nagi, "Disability Concepts Revisited," in *Disability in America*, Institute of Medicine (Washington: National Academy Press, 1991), pp. 313–315.

20. L. Liebman, "The Definition of Disability in Social Security and Supplemental Security Income," *Harvard Law Review* 89:5(March): 833–867.

21. *Americans With Disabilities Act.* 104, Stat. 327. July 26, 1990. A-7.

22. Nagi, "Disability Concepts Revisited," pp. 317–318.

23. M. Foucault, *Archaeology of Knowledge*, trans. A. M. Sheridan (New York: Harper Colophon, 1972), p. 46.

24. M. Foucault, "Two Lectures," in *Power/Knowledge: Selected Interviews and Other Writings, 1972–1977*, ed. C. Gordon (New York: Pantheon Books, 1980), pp. 93–94.

25. T. Nagel, "What Is It Like To Be a Bat?" *Philosophical Review* 83(1974): 435–450.

26. O. Sacks, "The Last Hippie," *New York Review of Books* 34:6(March 1992): 58.

27. I. Zola, *Missing Pieces* (Philadelphia: Temple University Press, 1982), p. 245.

28. The chief proponent of the view I call the "minority group model of disability" is political scientist Harlan Hahn (see reference below). I believe it consists of features that can be found in a loose family of conceptions of disability, even though there is a good deal of diversity within that family.

29. H. Hahn, "Theories and Values: Ethics and Contrasting Perspectives On Disability," in *Ethical Issues in Disability: Report of An International Conference: 1989*, ed. B. Duncan and D. E. Woods (World Rehabilitation Fund), p. 104.

30. Ibid.

31. ADA, A-5—A-6.

32. A. Caplan, D. Callahan, and J. Haas, "Ethical and Policy Issues in Rehabilitation Medicine," *The Hastings Center Report*, Special Supplement, August 1987: 145.

33. Ibid., p. 144.

34. D. Eddy. "The Challenge," *JAMA* 63(1990): 287–290.

35. O. W. Fiss, "Groups and the Equal Protection Clause," *Philosophy and Public Affairs* 5:2(Winter 1976): 123.

36. Hahn, "Theories and Values," p. 102.

37. E. Ezrahi, *The Descent of Icarus* (Cambridge, Mass.: Harvard University Press, 1990).

38. S. Shapin and S. Schaffer, *Leviathan and the Air Pump: Hobbes, Boyle and the Experimental Life* (Princeton: Princeton University Press, 1985), p. 339.

39. M. Minow, *Making All the Difference* (Ithaca: Cornell University Press, 1990).

40. W. Connolly, *Identity/Difference: Democratic Negotiations of Political Paradox* (Ithaca: Cornell University Press, 1991), p. 80.

9

THE SOCIAL COURSE OF CHRONIC ILLNESS
Delegitimation, Resistance, and Transformation in North American and Chinese Societies

ARTHUR KLEINMAN

> Our only hope will lie in the frail web of understanding of one
> person for the pain of another.
>
> JOHN DOS PASSOS
> DECEMBER 1940

Introduction

THE PURPOSE OF this essay is to explore social aspects of chronic illness and disability that do not figure significantly in the current biomedical discourse, or in that of bioethics, yet are features that anthropological studies and cross-cultural comparisons show to be influential and of considerable theoretical interest. In particular, I shall examine the place of three interpersonal processes—delegitimation, resistance, and transformation—in the social course of chronic pain and chronic fatigue syndromes. These processes mediate the embodiment of the moral context, and reciprocally provide the means by which alterations in the person who experiences chronic illness are projected outwardly into social space. I also intend to show that consideration of these broader social themes alters the way we conceive of the moral aspects of medicine.

Before these issues can be effectively examined, however, I first need to review an anthropological critique of the orthodox biomedical interpretation of chronic illness. That will establish the base for discussing an alternative, ethnographic theory of the relation between context and the body, a theory in which experience, including illness experience, is understood as a social field, or, in ethnographic parlance, a local world. From there, I shall illustrate the theory with examples from field research on chronic pain and fatigue syndromes in North America and

China. I draw upon these two illnesses because they are common chronic conditions and because patients who suffer from them often have frustrating experiences with health care, experiences that I believe crystalize problems patients with other chronic illnesses also undergo with health care in America. The conclusion will essay what is gained from the ethnography of chronic illness that can be applied to teaching, clinical care, and health policy. Is this ethnographic formulation of the social course of illness more valid than the biomedical formulation of the "natural history" of disease for configuring suffering as the object of medical inquiry and practice?

The Bias of Biomedicine

Central to the biomedical understanding of chronic illness—e.g., diabetes, asthma, schizophrenia, chronic fatigue syndrome, chronic pain syndrome—is the idea of a preprogrammed diathesis that exists inside the body independent of personal biography or context. That diathesis, it is held, outfolds into a standardized "natural" course. Diagnosis, treatment, and prognosis—the elemental tasks of the clinician—are said to be based upon knowledge of the "natural course" of the disease. So naturalized, the course of disease is envisaged as a trajectory that can be predicted and controlled. This orientation is central to the commitment to naturalism that biomedicine employs to separate medical from other conditions of human misery. Thus, disease is held to be a natural form of life that is different from poverty, political oppression, or social alienation; yet, each of these social problems has a physiology, so that, notwithstanding biomedicine's protestations to the contrary, the distinction must be viewed as a social construction with a particular purpose.

The commitment to naturalism is associated with other conceptual orientations fundamental to biomedicine (Lock and Gordon 1988). These include, *inter alia*, an extreme insistence on materialism as the grounds of knowledge, a focus on autonomous, individuated organisms, a requirement that single causal chains must be used to specify pathogenesis as structural flaws in the body's mechanical mechanism, and a predilection for powerful operations to fix that mechanism. Notable as well is an antivitalism, a discomfort with functional, processual dialectical thinking, and a rejection of teleology—disease is held to fall outside the intentionality and purposefulness of human constructions.

The biomedical definition of nature is determinatively physical. Nature can be (indeed, must be) understood, independent of perspective, representation, or context, as a "real" entity that can be "seen," a "thing" that stands beneath symptom and coping response as the generating source of pathognomonic pathology. Here we find the roots of the powerful program of reductionism through which medical students are trained to make biology visible as the ultimate reality, the fundamental substance behind complaints and illness narratives (Good 1994). All other orders of reality are suspect. There are, of course, alternative streams in biomedicine, and periodic attempts at formulating new directions aimed at reforming this paradigm. Nonetheless, what I have described is the mainstream position, an orthodoxy that is remarkably intolerant of alternatives.

This set of biases has indeed been successful as the raison d'être for the development and application of biochemical technologies which, for acute disease and its pathology, have led to so many impressive contributions. Yet, in the understanding of chronic illnesses and in the care of patients this reductionist program has proved to be disappointingly inadequate and even disabling for practitioners—a dehumanizing framework. Furthermore, much evidence has accumulated about the social roots and consequences of disease that simply cannot be accommodated within the cramped boundaries of the biomedical program. Reviewing merely a few findings challenges the biomedical bias while suggesting a more thoroughly social perspective.

Evidence for the Social Course of Illness

Evidence of the social causation of mortality and morbidity (Black 1980; House et al. 1989) and of the role of social factors in prevention (Mechanic 1994) is so very extensive that it is beyond the focus of this article. Findings that illustrate the powerful influence of social factors on the course and outcome of disorders are appropriate to consider here. Thus, with respect to disability, Yelin showed that perception of job satisfaction and quality of work relationships predicted better than radiologic methods which workers would leave the disabled list and return to work (Yelin et al. 1980). Pain patients may become chronically disabled owing to economic incentives and family and personal problems (Osterweis et al. 1987). Negative expressed emotion—e.g., critical comments made about the patient—in family members predicts worsening in the course of schizophrenia measured as rehospitalization over the subsequent period of six months or longer (Jenkins and Karno 1992)—a finding which has been extended to depression as well. The degree of perceived social support and stressful life-event changes among patients with chronic depressive and anxiety disorders have been found to exert a greater effect on outcome than treatment (Moos 1991). Indeed, interpersonal psychotherapy for major depressive disorder seems to be about as effective as antidepressant psychopharmacologic treatment for outcome (Klerman et al. 1984). In a study in the People's Republic of China, patients with neurasthenia, often associated with depression and anxiety, went on to recovery only after they had resolved a major social problem in workplace or family setting (Kleinman 1986). Although many other studies could be cited, these few should be sufficient to emphasize the idea that illness experiences have a decidedly social course. Economics, politics, and other macro-social structures, as well as micro-level work and family relationships, shape symptoms, pathology, and treatment choice and response.

Yet, if we take the notion of the social course of illness as seriously as it deserves, we also need to understand the social processes that mediate chronic illness as a moral career. The sociological idea of illness as a moral career implies that illness becomes a way of life and a means through which life choices and career plans are negotiated. Such a way of life, and of life advancement, is "moral" because the experience of illness is taken up in value commitments. In the sections that follow I will examine several such social processes in chronic illness. But to appreciate how they work, we first need to develop an ethnographic theory of the course of illness in particular social contexts that can later be used as a backdrop to the discussion of mediating processes.

Local Moral Worlds of Experience: The Ethnographer's Perspective

In a recent theoretical contribution, the work of continental phenomenologists (Bergson, Merleau-Ponty, Plessner, Gehlen), John Dewey (1957), William James (1981), ethnographers who emphasize experiential categories (e.g., Feld [1981], Jackson [1989]; Stoller [1989], Roseman [1990], and Desjarlais [1993]), and the French social theorist Pierre Bourdieu (1989) is drawn on to develop a conceptualization of experience as an intersubjective matrix of social transactions in local settings (Kleinman and Kleinman 1991). Experience so defined is a medium of communication and negotiation that is of overbearing practical relevance because something vital is at stake for the participants. Experience, then, is as much social process as subjective process. Indeed, the subjective and the social interpenetrate extensively. The self is dialogical (see Taylor 1989).

Experience, in this model, is the felt flow of the intersubjective medium. It is organized out of vital engagements and negotiations, under the pressure of what is perceived to be most pressingly relevant, in the daily struggles of social life. The cultural patterning of social experience occurs out of the coding of social action via linguistic, aesthetic, and other symbolic apparatuses. Cultural forms emerge, or are "realized," in the rhythms and rituals of everyday interactions, where the practical relevance of life plans and choices is worked out through conflict as much as consensus.

In this theoretical model, social experience connects institutional structures (kinship networks, class, and jural and political institutions) and systems of collective meaning that together constitute the moral order with body-self processes (see Bourdieu 1989). Thereby, the social world enters into cardiovascular, endocrinological, and neurobiological processes so as to pattern responses. In turn, bodily and self processes project into social space, bringing affect and embodied meaning to bear upon social life. In the section that follows, I will draw on this framework to analyze the contribution of such sociosomatic processes as mediators and transformers of chronic illness and disability.

Delegitimation, Resistance, and Transformation in the Social Experience of Illness

In a study of chronic pain patients in the Northeast of the United States, I examined the central role that delegitimation plays in their lives (Kleinman 1992). The analysis can be summarized as follows: pain patients frequently do not have extensive pathology. Their back pain and headaches are often said to be greatly in excess of the pathological findings in their nerves, muscles, bones, and joints (Osterweis et al. 1987). As a result, practitioners working in the biomedical framework are led to be suspicious about whether the pain is "real" (Scarry 1985). Faced with suspicion or even frank distrust, pain patients not surprisingly amplify their complaints to draw attention to their seriousness and to convince their caregivers that they are suffering. This dance of dramatized complaint and questioning response ultimately convinces practitioners that pain patients are "somatizers" who are exaggerating their illness experience for social or psychological reasons. (The problematic dynamic between doubt and amplification, however, can occur in any chronic illness.) Patients come to feel that their pain experience is delegitimated by their practitioners and by the psychosomatic labels those practitioners employ. There is an angry feeling of betrayal that may lead patients to discontinue care with a particular practitioner, to shop around for other caregivers, even to drop out of care—or, at the least, biomedical care—altogether. In turn, practitioners come to feel that pain patients are "problem" patients who do not want to get well. Mutual frustration is statistically associated with poor outcomes: addiction to narcotic analgesics; overuse of expensive and costly tests; polypharmacy; unnecessary surgery, which contributes to pathology; noncompliance; and patient and family dissatisfaction with care (Osterweis et al. 1987).

Seen from the perspective advanced here, the delegitimation that pain patients feel is a prime example of the social course of chronic illness. Under the regime of biomedicine these patients are accused of exaggeration or worse. Their symptoms are discounted, their illness experience is disaffirmed. They come to feel belittled; their sense of personal worth and self-efficacy is assaulted. The repercussions are extensive, for what is being disaffirmed is the entire network of coping transactions in which the illness is embedded. Delegitimation itself is a social process. What results is a pattern of care that is as threatening to the practitioner as it is demoralizing to the patient.

Another common "psychosomatic" disease of the current era—chronic fatigue syndrome—instantiates similar problems. The label is contested. Is it a "real" disease, i.e, a "physical" illness? Or is it the rediscovery of neurasthenia? Inasmuch as biomedicine eschews the validity of vitality as an essential aspect of being human, exhaustion and fatigue have no independent status as authentic problems in themselves, but rather are treated as consequences of other conditions: sleep disorders, depression, chronic infections, and so forth. Lacking the authenticity of independent status, this set of problems is as deeply suspect as is pain. When a contributing physical cause cannot be isolated in the work-up, the patient is relegated to a set of "psychosomatic" problems that delegitimate the complaint and the person. For the idea is that these problems are somehow less real, less serious, and possibly intentional. No wonder that patients struggle desperately to avoid the deeply discrediting description of a "stress-related," "psychosocial" or "psychosomatic" condition; or that patient advocacy groups insist that the disorder must be due to a virus and its immunological effects, in spite of negative findings. Moreover, disability status, with all its financial consequences, may not be granted or may be withdrawn owing to the inefficacy of psychosomatic labels.

Delegitimation occurs in the course of various chronic illnesses—especially those that are stigmatized (such as schizophrenia, depression, epilepsy) or not fully confirmed as legitimate (such as chronic pain syndrome, chronic fatigue syndrome, and many cases of Lyme disease and environmental allergies). It should not be thought of as an atypical untoward side effect of health care practices; but rather it needs to be seen as routine, a mainline process in care that is based upon the normative order of the larger society and its impact in the clinic and household. Delegitimation attacks the moral order of local worlds. It is illness-enhancing, and it also constrains the effect of treatment. Delegitimation intensifies suffering. Indeed, it re-creates suffering in a wholly other mode: illegitimate suffering. I would hypothesize that there may be a special physiology, a local one, for such a vexed social status.

In the course of research with chronic fatigue patients, it was discovered that 40 percent of patients, in a small but intensively followed sample of fifty chronic fatigue patients, most of whom were middle-class or working-class women, substantially transformed their lives. The illness label had provided them with an authoritative medical rationale to do so. Thereby, they changed exhausting, high-paced, high-pressured lifestyles into more leisured, protected havens in a frenetic world (Ware and Kleinman 1992). Thus, illness legitimated *social transformation* in local worlds that affected family members, friends, co-workers, and other significant parties in the "designated patient's" network. This may seem to be the obverse of the chronic pain example, but based on the dynamics of local worlds, patients with chronic pain and fatigue syndromes are vulnerable to either and perhaps both social experiences.

Chronic illness is not infrequently an occasion for local transformations. Families may divide or come together under the sign of disabling illness; jobs may be turned down or turned in; and different responses to community pressures may eventuate. The way patients and their circle come to deal with serious illness readily extends beyond the body-self to the moral world. Courage, forebearance, endurance, tragedy—terms easily applied to chronic illness—indicate the resonance between the social experience of suffering and the moral processes of everyday life. At times, the social resonance of suffering may extend much further yet into the social world, as when, for example, moral metaphors embodied in paradigmatic cases of illness serve to critique social structures and to inspire social reforms. Anorexia nervosa, with its association with a vicious commercial culture of thinness and sensuality in young women; post-traumatic stress disorders, with their relation to child abuse and political terror; Type A personality problems, which putatively correlate simultaneously with financial success and with coronary artery disease; substance abuse and AIDS among impoverished, unemployed inhabitants of inner-city slums—all may evoke such an ethos of criticism and reform (see Konner 1993; Littlewood and Lipsedge 1987; Farmer 1992; and Scheper-Hughes and Lock 1987).

A third process that mediates illness in its local context is *resistance*. Now, resistance can be understood in two rather different senses. Max Scheler (1971) defined resistance as the core experiential quality of reality. That resistance of the world to the life plans and chances of persons focuses attention on what is most at stake in reality: survival, success, failure, aspiration, suffering, death. Serious chronic illness is one of the most powerful examples of this type of existential resistance.

In its other sense, resistance has to do with resisting political oppression, an idea which, on first encounter, might seem rather remote from chronic illness experience. Yet, this form of resistance too can be found among the chronically ill, though it is not named as such. Noncompliance—the patient's intentional or non-intentional failure to follow the medical regimen—can sometimes represent resistance to medical authority. For the chronically ill, who are asked to follow strictly a greatly constraining change in diet and lifestyle, and to take expensive medicines with significant side effects or undergo dangerous technical procedures on a routine basis, the prescription takes on a moralizing image. "Do this! Don't do that!" From the mouth of an authoritarian caregiver, these messages can be felt as commands that cannot simply be accepted, say, by a North American patient with a strong sense of autonomy.

Medical anthropologists have noted the biphasic alternation in personal control throughout the course of illness and care (Alexander 1982). When patients' conditions are stable, they are expected to take responsibility for self-care; but when illnesses acutely worsen or treatment effects threaten the person just as seriously, then the patient (and family) are expected to release control to their professional caregivers. This alternation can be greatly problematic for patients, who often experience a no-win situation in which they are blamed for being too active when the illness worsens or too passive when the illness improves. Resistance to medical authority, to biomedical authoritarianism, may be a means of coping with the double bind.

The control exercised by biomedical institutions and their professionals over the illness experience easily slides over into control of life cycle and life plans (Freidson 1986). Patients and families not infrequently feel threatened by professional control, and find ways to resist it. Inasmuch as they frequently end up dealing with the representatives of insurance, disability, health care, and other bureaucratic institutions, resistance may become a form of conflict management with these agents of state authority. In this Weberian sense, sick persons and their circles resist the objectivizing rational-technical procedures of the bureaucracy on behalf of the deeply subjective sentiment, tradition, and ad hoc coping functions of the local moral order. In this sense, their resistance to bureaucratic definitions and procedures on behalf of the cussedly inexpedient and existentially inefficient quiddities of human conditions places the chronically ill at the forefront of the unequal power conflicts between the informal and formal sectors of the social world that are so momentous for human experience in our time. That resistance can turn into resentment, as Weber noted, also applies to the chronically ill. Resentment against authorities in the health professions who are seen as cold and indifferent is not uncommon. Nor is resentment against the tyranny of health in the popular images of the commercial media, where healthy young bodies are everywhere and the sick and disabled are invisible.

Another example of political resistance comes from China, where, at the close of the disasterous political turmoil of the Cultural Revolution, chronic symptoms of fatigue, pain, and disorientation, which were widespread, came to represent a disguised resistance and indirect criticism of victims against their victimizers in the apparatuses of power of the Communist State. Yet, this form of embodied resistance never developed into an effective form of responding to the dangerous actions of political authority, and it also frequently worsened the life conditions of patients (Kleinman and Kleinman 1991; Kleinman 1992).

The Cultural Significance of Suffering

I have attempted to show that chronic illness experience, notwithstanding biomedical models that insist on the contrary, takes a decidedly social course in local worlds which is not effectively described by biomedical models of physiology or by psychological models of individual coping strategies. Such experience is more validly assessed through interpersonal models of legitimation, delegitimation, relegitimation, and resistance which throw light on the social processes that mediate and transform the lives of patients and families. In the long course of living with a chronic illness, suffering has a great deal to do with the effects of symptoms and treatments on life contexts, life situations, life course, and life chances.

Professionals in the health care system are trained and, when in practice, are rewarded to take as the object of inquiry the disease and the individual's response to it. They frequently minimize the broad social scope of serious illness in the interpersonal space of everyday life. They also fail to engage the cultural significance of suffering as embodied moral critique and opportunity for social transformation and even transcendence. Yet, suffering is inseparable from these social processes, which are of importance to its experience and treatment. The chief issue for health care researchers and teachers, and especially for those concerned with the intersection of values and medicine, is to figure out strategies by which these aspects of suffering can be more validly understood and engaged in biomedicine and in the wider society.

Heretofore, the medical humanities and bioethics have overemphasized the individual experience of illness at the expense of its social and cultural sides. A historically informed ethnographic approach to suffering may offer a more promising means of engaging the questions raised here (see Kleinman 1988:227–257) That is, clinical care can be modeled on the practice of ethnography. The clinician can approach his or her task as if it involved entrance into a very different life world. The clinician's aim is to describe and interpret the nature of that world: what it feels like to live there. The clinician as ethnographer seeks to understand how meaning is made in the context of different values, social arrangements, and conflicts. The purpose is to appreciate the meanings of those living and dealing with the illness. The clinician's ethnographic orientation also means that the focus of understanding and intervention is the nexus of relationships within which an illness becomes a joint way of living in the world, a collective experience. At the same time, such an approach challenges the chief orientation of the Western tradition of addressing value issues in medicine through emphasis on the autonomy of the suffering person. I maintain that there is a role for anthropology, social history, and the other social sciences in shifting the object of inquiry to include the social processes of everyday local worlds which shape suffering in ways quite distinct from the usual individual psychological orientation of clinical and ethical approaches taken to this most human of conditions.

In closing, it may be useful to very briefly revisit the ethnographic approach to care to specify the process of description, interpretation, formulation, and engagement that I take to be a means of grounding care in the utterly human processes of everyday moral experience (Kleinman 1988:225–251]). The first step is the development of a relationship of empathic witnessing in which the health care provider works through distinctive perspectives on the illness experience: the patient's, that of key members of the social network, other providers', etc. The idea is to get at the felt experience as engaged in and understood by each of these participants. Central to this activity is elicitation of the story of sickness and treatment, and description of the effect of the illness on the local context of family, work, health care, disability system, and vice versa, their effect on the illness. Life history review and appreciation of the explanatory models of patient, family, and practitioners regarding etiology, symptomatology, pathophysiology, expected course, and what is feared in the illness experiences and the treatment may help facilitate engagement with the local world of interpersonal experience of suffering and coping. The emphasis is on the empathic witnessing by a positioned practitioner of patients and families who are also positioned in a local context, and not on methods of interrogating individuals as if they were free from the constraints of others. The practitioner, the patient, and the patient's family together plot a therapeutic narrative for treatment in which the practitioner seeks to meet them in the phenomenological space of the moral meaning of the illness as that which is vitally and ultimately at stake for them. Together they affirm the illness experience. Together they may look for delegitimation and resistance in order to come to terms with core moral questions concerning what is at stake.

Ultimately, the ethnography of care is meant to bring the meaning of illness in the lived experience of suffering to the center of practice. The process of existential affirmation of making meaning out of pain and suffering is meant to be a vital nexus, a deeply human engagement that should not be spelled out as a technical set of steps in a treatment manual. It is a process of mutual discovery. It is meant to remoralize the participants, including the practitioner, and to ground care in the essentials of their shared humanity: decency, mutuality, support, and existential engagement with the tests of usually difficult and often desperate experience. The engagement with suffering is the coming together of persons in a quest for understanding. It should not be one-sided; aspiration, hope, and transformation are to be affirmed as well. It is the ethnographic process itself—open-ended, uncertain, positioned interpretation and participation—that is humanizing. And, I believe this is as pertinent for the medical researcher and educator as for the practitioner and the patient.

Ultimately, the care of chronic illness turns on how endurance is understood in particular local worlds. Is it valued as a basis for transcendence? Is it a means of asserting solidarity? Or is it a deeply threatening reminder that technology and scientific rationality have their limits, that there are certain problems that cannot be fixed but must be lived through until the end? The practitioner, the patient, the family, and members of the wider network and local institutions form the context in which endurance is managed as the social process of living with an interminable affliction. The meanings of endurance need to move to the center of caregiving. Hope or destiny, transcendence or despair, these are the core moral issues in the social course of chronic illness that should be the focus for the existential work of the healer. That is why chronic illness has so much to teach us about the means and ends of human experience.

REFERENCES

Alexander, L. 1982. "Illness maintenance and the new American sick role." In N. Chrisman and T. Maretzki, eds., *Clinically Applied Anthropology*. Hingham, MA: D. Reidel (Kluwer). pp. 351–367.

Black, D. 1980. Inequality in health: A report. London: Department of Health and Social Security.

Bourdieu, P. 1989. "Social space and symbolic power." *Sociological Theory* 7(1): 14–24.

Desjarlais, R. 1993. *Body and Emotion: Yolmo Shamanism and the Calling of Lost Souls.* Philadelphia: University of Pennsylvania Press.

Dewey, J. 1957 [1922]. *Human Nature and Conduct.* New York: The Modern Library.

Farmer, P. E. 1992. *AIDS and Accusation: Haiti and the Geography of Blame.* Berkeley: University of California Press.

Feld, S. 1981. *Sound and Sentiment.* Philadelphia: University of Pennsylvania Press.

Freidson, E. 1986. *Professional Powers.* Chicago: University of Chicago Press.

Good, B. 1994. *Medicine, Rationality and Experience.* Cambridge: Cambridge University Press.

Good, M. J., P. Brodwin, B. Good, and A. Kleinman. 1992. *Pain as Human Experience: Anthropological Studies.* Berkeley: University of California Press.

House, J. S., K. R. Landis, and D. Umberson. 1989. "Social relationships and health." *Science* 241: 540–545.

Jackson, M. 1989. *Paths Toward a Clearing.* Bloomington: Indiana University Press.

James, W. 1981 [1890]. "The consciousness of self." In *The Principles of Psychology.* Cambridge, MA: Harvard University Press. pp. 279–379.

Jenkins, J., and M. Karno. 1992. "Expressed emotion among Mexican-descent families: Cultural adaptation of the method and principal findings." *American Journal of Psychiatry.*

Kleinman. A. 1986. *Social Origins of Distress and Disease: Depression, Neurasthenia and Pain in Modern China.* New Haven: Yale University Press.

———. 1988. *The Illness Narratives.* New York: Basic Books.

———. 1992. "Pain and resistance." In M. J. D. Good et al., eds., *Pain as Human Experience.* Berkeley: University of California Press.

Kleinman, A., and J. Kleinman. 1991. "Suffering and its professional transformation: Toward an ethnography of interpersonal experience." *Culture, Medicine and Psychiatry* 15(3): 275–301.

———. [In press.] Remembering the Cultural Revolution: Alienating pains and the pains of alienation. Presented at the panel on "Secret Histories: The Politics of Memory in China," Association for Asian Studies Annual Meeting, April 13, 1991, New Orleans. T. Y. Lin, W. S. Tseng et al., eds., *Mental Health in Chinese Culture.* Hong Kong: Oxford University Press.

Klerman, G. L., et al. 1984. *Interpersonal Psychotherapy of Depression.* New York: Basic Books.

Konner, M. 1993. *Medicine at the Crossroads: The Crisis in Health Care*. New York: Pantheon.

Littlewood, R., and M. Lipsedge. 1987. "The butterfly and the serpent: Culture, psychopathology and biomedicine." *Culture, Medicine, and Psychiatry* 11: 289–336.

Lock, M., and D. Gordon, eds. 1988. *Biomedicine Examined*. Hingham, MA: Kluwer.

Mechanic, D. 1994. "Promoting health: Implications for modern and developing nations." (Revised version of paper published in *Society* 27, 1990.) In L. Chen, A. Kleinman, and N. Ware, eds., *Health and Social Change in International Perspectives*. Cambridge, MA: Harvard University Press.

Moos, R. 1991. "Life stresses, social resources, and the treatment of depression." In J. Becker and A. Kleinman, eds., *Psychological Aspects of Depression*. Hillsdale, NJ: Lawrence Erlbaum Associates. pp. 187–214.

Osterweis, M., A. Kleinman, and D. Mechanic, eds. 1987. *Pain and Disability: Behavioral and Public Policy Perspectives*. Washington, DC: National Academy Press. (306 pp.)

Roseman, M. 1990. "Head, heart, odor, and shadow: The structure of the self, the emotional world and ritual performance among Senoi Temiar." *ETHOS* 18(3): 237–250.

Scarry, E. 1985. *The Body in Pain*. New York: Oxford University Press.

Scheler, M. 1971 [1928]. *Man's Place in Nature*. H. Meyerhoff, trans. New York: Noonday Press.

Scheper-Hughes, N., and M. Lock. 1987. "The mindful body." *Medical Anthropology Quarterly* 1: 6–81.

Stoller, P. 1989. *The Taste of Ethnographic Things: The Senses in Anthropology*. Philadelphia; University of Pennsylvania Press.

Taylor, C. 1989. *Sources of the Self: A Making of the Modern Identity*. Cambridge: Harvard University Press.

Ware, N., and A. Kleinman. 1992. "Culture and symptoms." *Psychosomatic Medicine* 54: 546–560.

Yelin, E., et al. 1980. "Toward an epidemiology of work disability." *Milbank Memorial Fund Quarterly/Health and Society* 58(3): 386–414.

10

THE ROLE OF THE RULES
The Impact of the Bureaucratization of Long-Term Care

MURIEL R. GILLICK

THE GERONTOLOGIST'S DREAM is a world in which "life is physically, emotionally, and intellectually vigorous until shortly before its close, when, like the marvelous one-hoss-shay, everything comes apart at once and repair is impossible."[1] Physicians continue to debate whether such a world is possible[2] and to argue about how much of the disability and chronic illness associated with aging is inevitable and how much is avoidable with good diet, exercise, and other preventive health measures.[3] Whatever good news the future may hold, the contemporary reality is that chronic disease and functional limitations (inability to perform many of the basic activities of daily living such as bathing, dressing, or, at a somewhat higher level, shopping or cooking) are widespread among the elderly. Recent data indicate that 12.0 percent of individuals aged 65–74 require assistance in at least one activity of daily living. This number rises to 22.4 percent for those aged 75–84 and soars to 39.8 percent for people 85 and over.[4] The striking frequency of functional limitations is not surprising when we observe that the most common medical disorders reported in the elderly include arthritis, hypertension, diminished hearing, heart disease, visual impairment, orthopedic impairment, arteriosclerosis, and diabetes.[5] These conditions are often associated with diminished mobility, problems with fine motor control, and difficulties interfacing with the outside world, all of which translate into the need for assistance in daily living.

Not only are chronic diseases widespread, resulting in extensive limitations of function, but the problems have been getting worse as the population ages.[6] The oft-cited statistics on the greying of America are most dramatic when they focus on the old old, those 85 and over: between 1960 and 1990 there was an impressive 88 percent increase in the population over 65 and a phenomenal 225 percent increase in those 85 and over. If the anticipated rate of growth of the elderly population occurs and if the current patterns of disability prevail, by the year 2040 there will be 13.1 million elderly who require assistance in daily living, including 5.2 million who live in nursing homes.[4]

The existence of a large cohort of elderly individuals who have significant functional limitations due to chronic disease and the predictions about their numbers in the future have generated interest in a variety of public health and public policy questions. In addition, there has been a surge of interest in seeking to maximize the functioning of the elderly individual from a medical point of view as geriatrics has gained in respectability as a subspecialty. An important adjunct to the medical and public health perspectives—some might argue a necessary prerequisite for meaningful health care or public policy—is an understanding of the experience of chronic illness and disability from the point of view of the elderly individual.

Influence on the Experience of Chronic Illness

The experience of chronic illness is determined to some extent by the particulars of the disease: a person who is paralyzed from a stroke has a different experience from that of an individual who is legally blind from diabetic retinopathy, who in turn has a different experience from a person with dementia who is becoming progressively more forgetful and paranoid. The experience of chronic illness is also shaped by the cultural context: the meaning of illness varies from society to society.[7] Within a given society, different ethnic groups have their own unique responses to sickness.[8] There is another major influence on the experience of illness, one to which little research or reflection has been devoted, and that is the caregiving system itself.

In the case of the elderly with chronic disease, the care that is provided is largely long-term care, as contrasted with the acute, episodic care that characterizes treatment of isolated episodes of illness. Long-term care has been defined as: "The provision of diagnostic, preventive, therapeutic, and supportive services to patients of all ages with a severe chronic disease or disability involving substantial functional impairment. The care, frequently of long duration, may be provided by a variety of health care professionals and other caregivers, formal and informal, in a variety of institutional and noninstitutional settings, preferably the home."[9] The institutions comprising the long-term care system can be expected to exert a powerful influence on the experience of illness and the quality of life of those with chronic disease.

I use institution here in the broadest possible sense to include all the loci of long-term care. Institutions, so defined, include the nursing home, the rehabilitation hospital, and the home. There are other institutions that deserve consideration as well, such as the hospice, retirement communities, life-care communities, and congregate (group) homes. By and large these are devoted to the terminally ill or to the very healthy elderly. I will therefore focus on the major institutions dedicated to the care of the chronically ill and ask how their structure affects both the quality of care (in the technical, medical sense) and the quality of life of those they serve.

The structure of long-term care institutions is determined by their historical development, by prevailing reimbursement systems, and by the government regulations under which they operate, as well as by the needs of their clients. Two major forces affecting long-term care institutions over the past twenty-five years have been the need to control costs and pressure for improving quality of care.

The Twin Themes of Cost and Quality

Since the introduction of Medicare and Medicaid in 1965, the federal government has footed the bill for a large fraction of long-term care. While that fraction has remained relatively constant, the number of individuals needing long-term care has increased dramatically. As a result, the total outlay by the government has risen substantially. In the realm of nursing home care, Medicaid pays 42 percent of the cost of care, Medicare about 2 percent, and other government programs an additional 4 percent (chiefly the Veterans Administration); however, the number of people in nursing homes nearly doubled between 1963 and 1977, and rose another 24 percent between 1980 and 1990.[4] In the home care arena, Medicare costs rose from $63 million in 1970 to $1.2 billion in 1982, and have continued to rise without substantial changes in the services covered. Medicaid costs for home health care rose from $15 million to $400 million over the same period.[10] These tremendous increases in expenditures have led both federal and state governments to seek to control costs by exerting tighter control over all long-term care institutions.

At the same time that government became more concerned about the rising costs of long-term care, the public has become increasingly concerned about quality of care. Investigations of nursing homes have repeatedly revealed inadequate care and abuse of residents, phenomena which have been reported on extensively by the media.[11] As a direct consequence of pressure by advocacy groups for the elderly, government regulation was gradually introduced into the long-term care system. Nursing homes, for instance, were only minimally regulated prior to the late 1960s. Detailed regulations governing skilled nursing facilities were not introduced until 1974. Eligibility for certification as a Medicare or Medicaid facility became contingent on adherence to these regulations. Concerns regarding the adequacy of care within both nursing homes and home care agencies persisted. After extensive work by health care professionals and consumer advocacy groups, the Omnibus Budget Reconciliation Act (OBRA) of 1987 was passed, which included general principles to govern new certification criteria. The Health Care Financing Administration (HCFA) then went on to develop detailed criteria for nursing homes (based on the recommendations of a study by the Institute of Medicine)[12] as well as revised certification standards for home health care agencies.[13]

As a result of the burgeoning regulations, long-term care institutions have been forced to alter many facets of their physical and administrative structure, their style of care, their fee system, and their admission policies. The nursing home industry, home health care agencies, and the rehabilitation hospitals that have been affected by the changes have protested what they regard as government intrusion into their domains. Physicians accuse government of infringing on their professional autonomy. While there has been a growing awareness of the bureaucratization of medicine, what is seldom analyzed is how this process is altering the experience of illness for the patient. The escalating regulation of health care affects all phases of the medical system. But in no area is this more dramatic than in long-term care, where the patient's encounter with the health care system is intense, frequent, and critical to his survival. It is to the long-term care institutions that we now turn, asking what effect their structure—in particular the rules governing their functioning—has on the patient's experience of illness.

The Nursing Home

There are currently close to 20,000 nursing homes in the United States.[14] These institutions are home to nearly 1.5 million Americans for an average of 2.9 years. The typical nursing home resident is an 86-year-old woman with multiple medical as well as psychosocial problems who is taking several medications.[15] More often than not, she entered the nursing home when her family and community agencies could no longer safely provide care for her because of her severe functional disabilities. Prior to her moving to the nursing home, she most likely had a longstanding relationship with a primary care physician.

When an elderly patient enters a nursing home, one of the first changes that affects her experience of illness is that she is likely to have a new physician. Doctors have a significant financial disincentive to care for nursing home patients: they are reimbursed poorly for nursing home visits, with minimal if any compensation for the travel time required to see a patient in the nursing home.[16] Nursing homes in general require that physicians come to the patients and will not tolerate an arrangement whereby a resident travels to his long-time physician's office for appointments. For older patients who are experiencing the dislocation of entering a nursing facility, the disruption entailed by simultaneously losing their physician may be considerable. This is particularly true if a major factor in coming to terms with chronic illness had been the knowledge that the patient had a partner in his primary care physician.

Once the resident settles into the nursing home, she will find that her new doctor makes visits in accordance with criteria established by Medicare or Medicaid, rather than by the physician, the patient, or the nature of the patient's illness. Seeking to ensure that patients are seen sufficiently frequently, current regulations call for a visit every 30 to 60 days.[17] For the medically stable resident, a visit every 30 days is excessive. The natural response of a physician who is compelled to see a patient without any medical justification is to make that visit perfunctory. The patient, who is accustomed to problem-driven office visits, may well feel she is being slighted. If an acute problem does arise, the nurse is usually the intermediary between the resident and the physician. For a mentally intact patient, relying on a nurse to interact with her physician undercuts the way she normally responds to her own symptoms.

Once the physician is called, he has several possible ways to proceed. He may prescribe treatment or diagnostic tests based on the nurse's assessment. He may choose to make a special trip to the nursing home although this is disruptive of his schedule, or he may decide to send the patient to the local hospital emergency room for evaluation. In practice, what this means for the resident is further loss of control over her medical care. Residing in a nursing home entails loss of autonomy in multiple domains: loss of control over when you have your meals, when you get up, and the activities in which you participate. To these must be added loss of control over the initiation of medical treatment. For the person who has successfully dealt with his chronic medical conditions by exercising control over his medical care, the result may be devastating. In addition, the individual may receive more technologically intensive management of his chronic conditions than he previously received or would prefer because his physician is not available to make a personal assessment and therefore relies on the assessment of emergency room physicians or on laboratory data.

Upon entering a nursing home, the individual quickly makes another discovery: her world is run by nurses. The name "nursing home" was not chosen by accident. Although an estimated 90 percent of hands-on care is actually provided by nurses' aides,[14] it is the nurses who supervise, organize, and otherwise shape the character of the nursing home. In general, while nurses and doctors may previously have played an important role in the lives of these patients and facilitated their coping with their illness, that involvement by nurses and doctors was typically episodic. In the nursing home, nurses are a constant feature of daily life. Each floor or unit has a nursing supervisor. The primary caregivers are nurses and nurses' aides, with social workers, physical therapists, occupational therapists, and other health care providers comprising the ancillary personnel. Some larger facilities have their own therapy staff, but the majority of nursing homes contract out for therapists as needed. This pattern underscores the fact that it is not the therapists or the social workers who create the structure of the nursing home: they are merely consultants who play a peripheral role. For the resident, the centrality of nursing in the home means that each day is built around fundamental nursing care needs such as medication administration, dressing changes, and taking vital signs.

In a hospital, the nursing and medical needs of the patients are so overwhelming that it is entirely rational to design an environment in which these needs are the primary focus. A widespread assumption is that nursing home residents likewise have numerous nursing care needs. Nursing home residents indisputably are dependent in many of the basic activities of daily living: the most recent survey available found 75 percent required assistance with dressing, 49 percent needed help with toileting, 71 percent had impaired mobility, 44 percent were at least sometimes incontinent, and 39 percent needed help with eating.[18] They usually have numerous chronic medical problems, and the data suggest that the nursing home population is getting progressively more dependent and sicker.[19] Nonetheless, the reason for institutionalization in most cases is not that there are medical conditions that required treatment that was unavailable at home; in most instances, the reason for institutionalization is the development of functional deficits (such as trouble walking or trouble dressing) or cognitive deficits that make remaining at home impossible without extensive assistance. Thus, however sick the nursing home residents are, they are often no sicker than their counterparts who live at home; they merely need more help. Nursing homes are not inherently nursing institutions.[20] It is in large measure because the financing of nursing home care has derived historically from Medicaid and to a lesser extent from

Medicare, both of which are medical programs, that nursing homes have been regarded as exclusively medical facilities.

Not only do regulations shape when, where, and by whom nursing home residents receive medical care, they also shape the kind of medical care they receive. In particular, the rules influence which medications patients get, what laboratory tests are ordered, and the style of medical practice.

The Regulation of Medications

Medications are relatively easy to regulate. It is clear from the physician's written orders exactly what drugs have been prescribed. It is also easy to come up with rules to govern the circumstances under which a medication is to be prescribed and to determine how a drug should be monitored. Thus drugs are an obvious target for regulation: they are undoubtedly prescribed in a less than optimal fashion by many physicians and they constitute a large part of the cost of medical care for the nursing home resident to third party payors. A prime example of drugs that are tightly regulated in the nursing home is antipsychotic or neuroleptic drugs, commonly used to sedate demented patients who exhibit agitation, violence, and other behavioral abnormalities. Several studies have indicated that nursing home patients are oversedated and overmedicated.[21] As a result, the recently implemented OBRA rules require that neuroleptics be used only for certain specified behaviors; these behaviors must be carefully documented in the medical record; the medication must be tapered and preferably discontinued after six months' time; and medication use on an "as needed" basis rather than on a fixed schedule is prohibited.[22]

Fixed criteria are perceived by physicians as antithetical to the concern that precipitated the regulations, namely, recognition that a physician with the requisite expertise must oversee the administration of such medication. If the medications can be prescribed as long as certain behaviors are identified, if blood levels are to be ordered at preordained intervals, and if the drugs are to be discontinued after a set period, then why is any medical sophistication necessary?

From the point of view of the patient, the regulations produce a series of unintended consequences. First, there is a disincentive to nursing homes to accept patients who already have a psychiatric diagnosis or are on particular medications, as these medications in and of themselves generate an extraordinary volume of paperwork. Second, there is increasing pressure on nursing homes to seek psychiatric consultation on patients as a means of satisfying the documentation requirements, to avoid being cited for excess medication use. Third, physicians may deliberately fail to give patients a medication they feel is indicated so as to avoid possible entanglements with regulatory agencies.

The Regulation of Laboratory Tests

The use of laboratory tests is also carefully monitored by the state regulatory authorities. In the acute care setting, the regulators suspect that physicians order too many laboratory tests. The presumption in the nursing home tends to be that doctors do not order enough tests. Again the regulations arise from a well-intentioned desire to protect from neglect defenseless older people with mental impairment. The rigid approach taken, however, mandates that laboratory tests be obtained on a regular basis, without regard for the particular circumstances of a given nursing home resident. Thus many nursing homes require that a diabetic patient have blood sugars drawn monthly, that patients on fluid pills have their kidney function checked every three months, and that a panel of screening blood tests be obtained annually. There is little if any data on which to base recommendations for the frequency of laboratory testing in nursing home residents.[23] Many are extremely elderly and the goal of therapy is often to optimize function and maintain comfort, not to tightly control disease. Frequency of testing can readily be individualized: a person who has been on a stable dose of medication for years with good control of blood sugar may do fine with a sugar measurement once every six months. It may be wiser to monitor blood sugar selectively if there is a fluctuation in weight or at times of acute illness or poor nutrition rather than to seek to treat diabetes by an algorithm.

The regulations governing nursing homes often lead to the resident's acquiring a new physician, and to evaluation of acute medical problems in an emergency room or by a panel of laboratory tests rather than by a personal examination by the physician; the regulations contribute to the medicalization of nursing homes, and to rigid and perhaps arbitrary usage of medications and tests. This is not meant to be a comprehensive list of the effects of the bureaucratization of nursing home care, but rather a sample of some of the ways in which the rules affect the lives of the elderly with chronic illness.

Most older people—95 percent at any given time—do not live in nursing homes. Those living in the community, like their counterparts in the nursing home, have rising levels of dependency as a function of age. While approximately 80 percent of the help required by older people living at home is provided by family members,[24] the remainder devolves upon home care agencies. It is to this component of long-term care that I now turn.

The Home

An estimated 75 percent of frail and disabled older individuals receive long-term care in the community.[25] To provide this care, an enormous number of home care agencies have appeared on the American scene: climbing from 2,000 in 1966, when Medicare and Medicaid began funding home care, to over 10,000 in 1987.[26] These agencies offer an array of services: part-time nursing, physical therapy, occupational therapy, and social work services, as well as home health aides. In addition, some states have obtained special waivers to expand long-term care services to include case management, adult day care, and respite care. Assorted other services are available in many areas, such as home delivered meals through the Older Americans Act of 1965. Not surprisingly, home care is the fastest growing segment of the health care industry.

Home is preferable to institutional care for most elderly people precisely because it affords the privacy and the autonomy that are so often threatened in an institution. Yet those elderly who have chronic illnesses and are in need of assistance from the medical care system for their very survival find that the current structure of long term care affects their experience of illness even when they remain at home.

Home Care Regulations Favor Acute Illness

The most fundamental way in which home care regulations affect the elderly with chronic illness is through the denial of chronic illness as worthy of Medicare support. Quite simply, the Medicare program defines itself as an acute care insurance policy, and refuses to pay for medical or other services that help maintain the chronically ill. There are several notable exceptions; the dialysis program, funded since 1972 under Medicare, guarantees dialysis treatment indefinitely to all patients with chronic renal failure; the hospice program, a special Medicare benefit since 1983, provides services of a supportive nature to patients who are certified by their physicians as having a life expectancy of six months or less; Medicare will permit a visiting nurse to give monthly B12 shots as treatment for pernicious anemia to a patient with an unequivocal diagnosis of this disorder, as long as that person is homebound. But Medicare in general is explicit that visiting nurses, physical therapists, and home health aides supplied through the Visiting

Nurse Association are justified only if the patient is deemed medically unstable.[27] Typically, the nurse may make a handful of visits after an acute hospitalization or the development of a new medical problem. Once there are no dressings to be changed, no modifications of medications or dosages, the nurse pulls out.

The insistence on providing service only for new, acute problems devalues the role of maintenance treatment in chronic illness. Stroke patients complain that once physical therapists, speech therapists, and occupational therapists terminate their services, they begin to deteriorate. They often feel—and their therapists concur—that they are more likely to maintain their gains if they are in a long-term rehabilitation program.[28] The regulations specify that once a patient has reached a plateau, once he is not making further progress, he is no longer eligible for services. The same applies to an insulin-requiring diabetic who, after extensive education in diet and home glucose monitoring, achieves a level of stability in blood sugars. That patient no longer is eligible for home services.

Regulations Affecting Physician Services

As long as the patient is homebound, he is allowed to have physician office visits but not to be monitored at home by a visiting nurse unless his medical condition is stable. Medicare will pay for him to go to the physician's office via ambulance if he is truly homebound, at a cost of approximately $175 each way, but will not pay the $50 for a nurse to make a home visit.

The chronically ill elderly patient may decide simply to travel to a physician's office by ambulance, he may choose to pay out-of-pocket for home care services, or he may decide that if the Medicare program does not choose to cover certain services they must be unnecessary. An alternative would appear to be for the physician to make house calls. While Medicare reimburses physicians for house calls, the fees set by Medicare for physician home visits are lower than those for nurses.[16] In addition, Medicare requires that physicians provide supervision of any home care plan drawn up by community agencies, but does not permit billing for this supervisory or case management service. Medicare has recently acknowledged that the telephone calls to family members and to the panoply of community agencies involved in supporting home care patients are time-consuming and has supplied these services with billing codes. To date, however, there is no reimbursement provided for any of the codes.[26] The result of this systematic bias is that the number of house calls has been steadily declining: the most recent surveys indicate that home visits constitute considerably less than one percent of all patient visits.[29]

Because there is a need for home care by physicians—in fact, an increasing need as the population ages and other pressures work to keep a larger fraction of the elderly out of institutions—programs have arisen to meet this need. In general, these programs have been set up by teaching hospitals as a means of giving medical students, internal medicine and family practice residents, and geriatrics fellows experience in the care of the elderly. The Boston University Home Medical Service, in existence since the nineteenth century, has for many years been the principal vehicle for teaching geriatrics to fourth-year medical students.[30] The Montefiore Housecalls program, started in the 1940s, incorporates house officers into the ranks of visiting physicians.[31] While a number of additional house call programs have been set up as a means of exposing residents in family practice and internal medicine to geriatrics in general and to home visits in particular, there are powerful economic forces mitigating against their establishment: the hospital sponsoring the service is not allowed to bill for physician visits unless a senior, attending physician is physically present at the home along with the resident physician. This is in contradistinction to outpatient clinic visits, in which the patient is billed for an office visit even if she is seen only by a resident physician, as long as the attending physician is available for supervision. Thus, despite the requirement that family practice residents devote curricular time to home visits, and despite the recommendation that internal medicine residents also have such experience, according to the most recent survey only 34 percent of family practice programs and virtually no internal medicine programs included any time for house calls.[26] A valuable training and service opportunity has been lost, at least in part because of the restrictive Medicare regulations.

Retrospective Disallowal of Home Care Services

Yet another example of the adverse consequences of the bureaucratization of home care arises not so much from the regulations themselves as from their implementation. As the Health Care Financing Administration (HCFA) has no direct way of assessing the quality of home care services, the agency decides whether or not to reimburse for services rendered based on whether there was adequate documentation of the need for the interventions and whether the patient qualified in accordance with Medicare guidelines. This approach has had a profound impact on the recipients of home care in two ways. First, nurses, therapists, and social workers employed by home care agencies are taught how to document what they do in language acceptable to the Medicare reviewers, and subsequently spend a substantial part of their time engaged in extensive documentation. Since these employees have a fixed time commitment to the home care organization for which they work, the time spent on learning techniques of documentation and on carrying out the paper work translates into poor staff morale and less time for direct patient care.[32] Second, because Medicare reviewers became known for frequent retrospective denials of payment, many agencies have chosen a very strict interpretation of the regulations so as to minimize their losses.[33] To receive home care services from a Visiting Nurses Association (VNA), for example, a patient must be homebound. This has been defined by the HCFA as meaning that the patient "needs assistance" to leave home, has a medical problem rendering it unsafe to leave home, or effectively only leaves home to receive medical care.[28] To avoid the risk of not being paid for services already provided, VNAs in some cases chose to interpret the requirement of "homebound" status to deem ineligible an 85-year-old patient with severe arthritis because she was able to walk a distance of ten yards with her walker. A successful suit against the Department of Health and Human Services on the grounds of capricious retroactive denials may lead to improvement in the future. For now, home health care agencies continue to devote extensive resources to documentation and to assume a defensive posture vis-à-vis the government, resulting in less care for the chronically ill elderly.

The patchwork of legislation, codes, and certification criteria that govern the operation of agencies providing home health care has the principal result of restricting who can get help and how much can be gotten. At another level, the regulations fail to acknowledge the seriousness of chronic illness. By setting up barriers to physicians making house calls and by promoting lack of continuity in nursing services, they make it difficult for the elderly to cope with chronic illness. In the extreme, the inadequacy of home care may result in abandonment of the home in favor of the nursing home.

The Rehabilitation Hospital

The institution that often plays a pivotal role in determining whether an elderly individual who has been acutely ill will go home from a hospital or enter a nursing home is the rehabilitation hospital. Strictly speaking a short-stay facility, the rehabilitation hospital typically cares for patients in the subacute phase of a chronic illness, for periods of time measured in weeks rather than days. It is therefore useful to think of the rehabilitation hospital as lying along the spectrum of long-term care. A patient who has had a stroke, for instance, and is not ill enough to remain hospitalized but not well enough to go home, and who is thought to have the potential for further recovery, may be a candidate for intensive rehabilitation. A patient who breaks a hip and qualifies for a postoperative stay at a rehabilitation center stands an excellent chance of being able to return home. While prolonged post-fracture rehabilitation is not essential to a successful return home, there is evidence that the shorter the period of rehabilitation the greater the likelihood of admission to a nursing home. One study demonstrated that after the introduction of prospective payment for acute hospital care, length of hospitalization was dramatically reduced, with a concomitant diminution in physical therapy during the hospitalization and a resultant 50 percent increase in the proportion of patients discharged to a nursing home.[34]

Inpatient rehabilitation programs—either in a free-standing rehabilitation hospital or in a special rehabilitation unit of a general hospital—are typically designed for individuals who have lost function in several domains and who can be expected to benefit from some combination of physical therapy, occupational therapy, and speech therapy. While certain kinds of medical problems addressed by rehabilitation hospitals, such as head trauma and spinal cord injury, occur most commonly in younger individuals, the majority of the problems encountered by rehabilitation facilities are diseases of the elderly. Seventy-five percent of all strokes occur in people over sixty-five, limb amputations because of peripheral vascular disease or diabetes are performed principally in the elderly, and hip fractures, another major source of referrals to the rehabilitation hospital, occur almost exclusively in older people.[35]

The Effect of Admissions Criteria

Rehabilitation hospitals are governed by their own unique set of operating rules. Each rehabilitation hospital decides whether or not a given individual qualifies for admission—usually based on a screening by a nurse, who presents her view of the facts of the case to an admissions director or committee. In an acute care hospital, the decision to admit a patient is made by emergency room physicians or the patient's primary physician, or some combination of the two. The patient needs to be ill enough to require "hospital-level care"—care that could not be provided at home or in a nursing home, usually involving therapy such as intravenous medications or a respirator or a surgical procedure. However, there is a certain amount of discretion that can be exercised by the physician acting as the patient's advocate. For instance, a variety of infections (including cellulitis, pneumonia, and kidney infections) can be treated either intravenously or orally. If the patient and physician feel it would be beneficial to enter the hospital, the intravenous route can be chosen so as to justify the need for "hospital-level care." In the case of the rehabilitation hospital, those deciding on admissions are not the patient's advocate. The primary care physician can argue on behalf of the patient through the medium of the medical record, but the physician does not make the decision. Moreover, in the case of the acute care hospital, a physician on the staff of the hospital can decide to admit a patient if it his judgment that hospitalization is indicated, regardless of Medicare rules. At worst, Medicare can "disallow" the admission—jargon for refusal to pay. The patient can, nonetheless, for a fee, receive care. Moreover, there is an appeals process, so that if the patient and the physician disagree with Medicare's claim that the hospitalization is unnecessary, they can appeal the ruling. In the case of the rehabilitation hospital, there is no patient advocate on the admissions committee, and there is no appeals process.

There is another distinctive characteristic of the rehabilitation hospital's admissions process. Patients are selected based on whether it is felt to be virtually certain that they will benefit from therapy. It is not enough to have a qualifying diagnosis such as a stroke or a hip fracture. It is not enough to have a condition that would benefit from physical therapy, occupational therapy, or speech therapy. The rehabilitation hospitals wish to be as certain as possible that the patient will progress sufficiently so as to be able to return home within two to ten weeks. They do not wish to be left with patients who are unable to go home and need placement in a nursing home, a process which can take time.[36] Given the impossibility of making such predictions with certainty, the rehabilitation facility can only achieve this goal by periodically rejecting patients who would in fact benefit. If the acute care hospital acted in an analogous fashion, it would deny admission to all who had a reasonably high probability of dying despite aggressive treatment. Since 61 percent of all deaths occur in the hospital,[37] acute care hospitals would turn away a significant proportion of the patients they currently see fit to admit.

From the point of view of elderly patients with multiple chronic illnesses, the restrictive admission policies of the rehabilitation hospitals translate into a formidable barrier to entry. The 65-year-old with a hip fracture and no underlying medical problems is a much safer bet than the 85-year-old who was barely making it at home before she had a stroke and who will need a complicated care plan to remain independent in the community if she manages to recover at least partially from her neurologic deficits. The 80-year-old with a recent heart attack who was agitated and confused while in the coronary care unit and who is gradually building up her strength does not look very attractive to the rehabilitation hospital. She tires easily and gets discouraged frequently, leading the rehabilitation hospital screening committee to question whether she is sufficiently motivated to profit from an intensive rehabilitation environment.

Effect of a Separate Rehabilitation Staff

Once a patient successfully overcomes the admissions hurdle, he is uprooted from both his home and the acute care hospital to enter a new program in a new place. A few hospitals have their own rehabilitation ward or wing. In most cases, however, the patient must start all over with new physicians and new therapists in a physically foreign location. The patient's primary physician is usually not on the staff of the rehabilitation facility, so that medical problems that develop will be dealt with by a physician who does not know the patient—or, since the rehabilitation hospital typically has limited in-house medical coverage and limited laboratory and x-ray facilities, dealt with by shipping the patient back to the acute care hospital once more. For elderly patients, who commonly find changes in surroundings disorienting, such upheaval is distressing and may be deleterious to their recovery.[38] This is not merely a theoretical concern: one study of patients admitted to a geriatric inpatient rehabilitation unit found that there was a significant need for ongoing medical intervention, with 12 percent of patients transferred back to the acute general hospital.[39]

The Effect of the Three-Hour Rule

The actual day-to-day operation of all inpatient rehabilitation facilities is shaped by HCFA regulations. In an effort to be sure that rehabilitation hospitals operated efficiently, HCFA decided in 1982 that inpatients must receive at least three hours a day of physical therapy and occupational therapy five days a week, with a slightly reduced requirement on weekends. Institutions that fail to comply with these rules risk losing the waiver that exempts them from prospective payment and risk denial of payment. Interestingly, a study of the effects of the three-hour rule found that the requirement produced neither a decrease in length of stay nor improvement in functional status at the time of discharge. It did disclose a significant increase in complaints of overwork and fatigue, as well as a marked increase in the cost per patient.[40]

The effect of Medicare regulation of rehabilitation hospitals on elderly individuals with chronic illness is twofold. First, there are major barriers to entry, which have had particularly disastrous consequences since the introduction of prospective payment for acute care hospitals and the ensuing shorter length of stay for elderly patients. Second, for those patients who are accepted into a rehabilitation hospital, the treatment may be needlessly grueling.

Reforming the Long-Term Care System

From the patient's perspective, there is a complicated array of regulations that affect the experience of chronic illness. Although the regulations are intended to improve quality of care, patients often find that the rules irrationally decrease their access to care, prevent continuity of care, disrupt their lives by excessively medicalizing their existence, and alter the way their doctors prescribe medications and order tests. How can the long-term care system be reformed so as to truly optimize the function of the individual, as it is supposed to do?

Critiques of the long-term care system and proposals for reform are not new.[41] They typically focus either on expanding coverage, so that nursing home care, for instance, would be paid for by long-term care insurance,[10] or on developing a single, comprehensive system of care to replace the numerous existing overlapping agencies.[42]

Such reforms are important. First, they would protect the elderly from impoverishing themselves to secure quality care in their old age. The yearly cost for nursing home care ranged from $20,000 to $45,000 in 1990,[43] resulting in the majority of Americans spending down their resources and becoming Medicaid-eligible within months of entering a nursing home.[44] Second, creating a single payor for all long-term care services would abolish the prevailing tendency of government programs to cost-shift. The concern that patients might linger in a rehabilitation hospital while awaiting a nursing home bed, for example, which I argued discourages rehabilitation hospitals from accepting risky patients, reflects the fact that the rehabilitation hospital is paid by Medicare while the nursing home is paid by Medicaid. If both institutions were reimbursed by the same source, there would be no reverse competition (aspiring to find another party to service your client). Similarly, Medicare has no incentive to pay for ongoing home medical services even if the alternative to adequate home care is nursing home care: if an individual enters a nursing home, she will most likely either pay privately or be covered by Medicaid. From the point of view of Medicare, there is actually an incentive to favor institutional care over home care so as to permit cost-shifting. A public plan covering medical and social long-term care services, ranging from homemaking and home-delivered meals to nursing and physical therapy, would free the providers of care to give care based on need rather than eligibility. Third, reorganization of the long-term care system has the potential to decrease costs by increasing overall efficiency, by avoiding duplication of services, and by reducing administrative waste.[45]

The proposed reforms would go a long way toward a more efficient and comprehensive system, but they would not address the adverse effects of the plethora of regulations on the lives of individuals in nursing homes, in rehabilitation hospitals, or at home. The source of this problem is that the regulations which are supposed to promote quality of care are grounded in an anachronistic philosophy of quality assurance.

Quality Assurance in the Medicare Program

The approach to quality assurance endorsed by Medicare and Medicaid is based on what has been called the bad apples theory.[46] Poor quality, in this view, arises from inadequate motivation, sloth, or ignorance. A search for deviant providers will uncover those individual caregivers or institutions who are deficient. Moreover, the alleged deficiencies can be remedied by penalizing the malfeasants. In the case of long-term care institutions, whether nursing homes, home care agencies, or rehabilitation hospitals, this philosophy is translated into practice via a system of inspections which are required for certification. For the institution to be certified, and hence to receive government reimbursement for services rendered, it must adhere to certain easily measurable standards for the delivery of care. An additional way in which the government philosophy is implemented is by retrospective denial of payment. Rather than threatening to decertify a long-term care institution—which from a practical point of view would entail closing it down—the government can also threaten to not pay the institution. Analogous to the inspectors involved in the certification process are the reviewers who decide whether or not to authorize reimbursement for long-term care services.

It is clear that some kind of regulation is desirable—many abuses have been rectified since the intensification of regulation over the past twenty years. In particular, assessing such things as adherence to fire and sanitation codes, the nutritional adequacy of institutional food, and the availability of adequate numbers of appropriately trained staff lend themselves to the methods of government regulators. The need for regulation of long-term care in the United States has been recognized since the time when care was first provided outside the family, for pay rather than for love. The public almshouses of the nineteenth century as well as private old-age homes were regularly inspected by state authorities.[47] What must be questioned is the contemporary regulatory process. We must cease to accept without challenge "the prevailing world of the regulators [in which] inspection is adversarial, measurement is for purposes of punishment, not learning; and the gathering and publication of performance data [it is assumed] will somehow induce otherwise indolent providers to improve their care and their efficiency."[48]

Alternative Strategies for Achieving Quality

The principal approach to quality assurance other than the restrictive, punitive regulatory model espoused by government is total quality management (TQM), or continuous quality improvement (CQI). This approach derives from industry, where it has proved effective in guaranteeing quality of production line outputs. Rather than depending on inspections, TQM advocates continuous on-the-job quality assessment by all those involved in production. TQM entails breaking down barriers between staff, eliminating work quotas, adopting strong leadership, and offering in-service education. In addition to its successes in the factory, TQM has been useful in optimizing the functioning of other highly stereotyped processes such as the flow of patients in a physician's office.[49] How useful the fundamentally statistical approach of the original TQM theory will be in promoting high-quality medical care within long-term settings (or in other medical sites) remains to be determined.

A crucial facet of TQM which is relevant to the long-term care system is the internal monitoring of care. In contrast to the current regulatory system, a new framework for regulation must start with the identification of problems and an analysis of why they exist. It must develop educational programs and structural changes within the institution, as well as a system of individual incentives to produce change. To quote the head of a large chronic care facility: "Quality . . . ought to be more than conformance to arbitrary standards. It ought to be more than visiting armies of inspectors conducting orgies of measurement. Rather, quality should—indeed, must—be something that it is internally driven. It must embody a strategy for (1) discovering what is truly important to the infirm elderly who are in the care of the institution, their families, and the community; and (2) effecting ongoing, incremental, systematic improvements in the delivery of services to these various constituencies."[48]

Internal regulation, by itself, will probably be inadequate to assure quality care for the elderly with chronic illness. There is a long history of peer review in the acute care hospital that proved inadequate to produce meaningful change. Complementing a new system of comprehensive internal control should be a new kind of external regulation. The job of the external authorities in such a system would be to check whether each branch of the long-term care system was successfully implementing its own internal process of self-evaluation and self-correction, rather than actually doing the regulating.[50] Such an approach is predicated on the observation that despite the tremendous progress in the field of quality assurance,[51] it remains difficult to specify, using readily measurable critera, what constitutes quality care in the long-term setting. While an external agency may not be able to determine whether optimal care is being delivered, that agency will be able to assess whether the institution has in operation an assessment process that both identifies problems and establishes remedies.[50] This dual approach to quality assurance could be broadly applied to a variety of medical settings. With the development of large group practices and health maintenance organizations, there is an opportunity to develop more effective ongoing education, feedback, and standard-setting within medical institutions. The development of a combined system of internal and external regulation in the long-term care arena will be more complex.

Implications for Long-Term Care

In the case of the nursing home, significant structural modifications will be necessary to shape an effective internal monitoring process. Nursing homes remain highly decentralized, precisely the feature that has been cited as the historical reason that American medicine evolved more extensive external regulation than any other Western country.[50] Either nursing homes will need to expand so as to be able to hire their own medical staff (as presently is done in a handful of facilities), or groups of institutions will need to form loose conglomerates and require admitting physicians to participate in quality assurance activities and monitoring activities, along with nurses, nurses' aides, and other staff.

Each nursing home needs to develop its own solution to the problems that precipitated regulation. Strategies to ensure that residents receive adequate physician evaluation of medical problems, or to guarantee that residents are not needlessly restrained or sedated could be devised by a group comprised of staff members (nurses, aides, and administrators), physicians, family members of residents, and, when feasible, the residents themselves. This group would be forced to grapple with the issues of quality and cost control and to be sensitive to the idiosyncracies of the home that might warrant unique, institution-specific solutions. The presence on the committee of individuals who are not employed by the nursing home would itself promote quality by guaranteeing that outsiders were frequently on-site, informally surveying care. Ideally, the home would obtain waivers from the state regulatory agencies permitting substitution of local solutions for the prevailing approaches to quality control. Such a communitarian approach would allow diversity to flourish and would give each home a greater stake in delivering top quality care because the employees would be implementing a program of their own design.

In home care, each organization needs to develop a mechanism for assessing the skills of nurses and therapists in the field. Utilization of home care agencies as training sites for nursing schools might afford an opportunity to expose staff to seminars and lectures provided by the affiliated educational institution as a quid pro quo for clinical teaching. Home care agencies may need to employ their own physicians to provide primary care for patients, to serve as a resource for nurses, and to help integrate home and hospital care.[52]

In the realm of the rehabilitation hospital, research is needed to determine just who benefits from rehabilitation and what kind of programs are most likely to be effective. Each unit within a rehabilitation facility should establish its own quality assurance process.[53] Collaboration by geriatricians (internists and family physicians specializing in the care of the elderly) and physiatrists (specialists in rehabilitation medicine) could result in a creative system of internal regulation. The efficacy of these systems for monitoring and self-improvement could readily be demonstrated to external review agencies.

Conclusion

I have argued that it is important to take a "micro" as well as a "macro" look at reforming the long-term care system. It is essential not only to address issues of access, efficiency, and comprehensiveness, but also to look at the effect of the current morass of government regulations on the experience of the elderly people with chronic illness who depend on long-term care. A series of examples of the extant regulations in three long-term care settings—the nursing home, the home, and the rehabilitation hospital—reveal the ways in which the rules, while intended primarily to assure quality of care and to control costs, are often detrimental to the well-being of those they are supposed to serve. The source of this paradox, I suggest, is the philosophy undergirding the regulatory system. Only by radically altering the nature of the regulatory system can we hope to develop long-term care institutions whose impact on the elderly with chronic illness is decisively positive.

REFERENCES

1. Fries, J. "Aging, Natural Death, and the Compression of Morbidity." *N Engl J Med* 1980; 303: 130–135.

2. Schneider, E. and Brody, J., "Aging, Natural Death, and the Compression of Morbidity: Another View." *N Engl J Med* 1983; 309: 854–856.

3. Rowe, J. and Kahn, R. "Human Aging: Usual and Successful." *Science 1987*; 237: 143–149.

4. Schick, F. and Schick, R., eds. *Statistical Handbook on Aging Americans.* Phoenix, Arizona: Oryx Press, 1994.

5. US Senate, Select Committee on Aging. Aging America: Trends and Projections. Washington, D.C., 1984.

6. Verbrugge, L. "Longer Life but Worsening Health. Trends in Health and Mortality of Middle-Aged and Older Persons." *Mil Mem Fund Q* 1984; 62: 475–519.

7. Kleinman, A., Eisenberg, L., Good, B. "Culture, Illness and Cure. Clinical Lessons from Anthropologic and Cross-Cultural Research." *Ann Intern Med* 1978; 88: 251–258.

8. Zborowski, M. "Cultural Components in Responses to Pain." In E. G. Jaco, ed. *Patients, Physicians, and Illness.* New York: Free Press, 1958, pp 16–30.

9. Somers, A. "Insurance for Long-Term Care. Some Definitions, Problems, and Guidelines for Action." *N Engl J Med* 1987; 317: 23–29.

10. Health and Public Policy Committee. American College of Physicians. "Financing Long-Term Care." *Ann Intern Med* 1988; 108: 279–288.

11. Vladeck, B. *Unloving Care: The Nursing Home Tragedy.* New York: Basic Books, 1980.

12. Institute of Medicine. *Improving the Quality of Care in Nursing Homes.* Washington, D.C.: National Academy Press, 1986.

13. Winograd, C. and Pawlson, G. "OBRA 87—A Commentary." *J Amer Geriatr Soc* 1991; 39: 724–726.

14. Ouslander, J. "Medical Care in the Nursing Home." *JAMA* 1989; 262: 2582–2589.

15. Libow, L., Starer, P. "Care of the Nursing Home Patient." *N Engl J Med* 1989; 321: 93–96.

16. Meiches, R. "Medicare Guidelines for Physician Reimbursement of Nursing Home Patients." *American Geriatrics Society Newsletter* 1991; 20(1): 1.

17. American Hospital Association, Section for Aging and Long-Term Care Services. Final Rule on Medicare/Medicaid: Requirements for Long-Term Care Facilities. September, 1991.

18. National Center for Health Statistics. Health, United States, 1987. DHHS Pub. No. (PHS) 88-1232. Washington, D.C.: US Government Printing Office, 1988.

19. Shaughnessy, P., Kramer, A. "The Increased Needs of Patients in Nursing Homes and Patients Receiving Home Health Care.'" *N Engl J Med* 1990; 322: 21–27.

20. Gillick, M., "Is the care of the chronically ill a medical prerogative?" *N Engl J Med* 1984; 310: 190–193.

21. Beers, M., Avorn, J., Soumerai, S., Everitt, D., Sherman, D., Salem, S. "Psychoactive Medication Use in Intermediate-Care Facility Residents." *JAMA* 1988; 260: 3016–20.

22. Garrard, J., Makris, L., Dunham, T., Heston, L., Cooper, S. et al. "Evaluation of Neuroleptic Drug Use by Nursing Home Elderly under Proposed Medicare and Medicaid Regulations." *JAMA* 1991; 265: 463–467.

23. Levinstein, M., Ouslander, J., Rubenstein, L., Forsythe, S. "Yield of Routine Annual Laboratory Tests in a Skilled Nursing Home Population." *JAMA* 1987; 258: 1909–15.

24. Brody, E. " 'Women in the Middle' and Family Help to Older People." *The Gerontologist* 1981; 21: 471–480.

25. Keenan, J., Fanale, J., "Home Care: Past and Present, Problems and Potential." *J Amer Geriatr Soc* 1989; 37: 1076–83.

26. Keenan, J., Fanale, J., Ripsin, C., Billows, L. "A Review of Federal Home-Care Legislation." *J Amer Geriatr Soc* 1990; 38: 1041–48.

27. Steel, K. "Home Care for the Elderly: The New Institution." *Arch Intern Med* 1991; 151: 439–442.

28. Reed, R., Geretz, M., Winograd, C. "Expanded Access to Rehabilitation Services for Older People. An Urgent Need." *J Amer Geriatr Soc* 1990; 38: 1055–56.

29. Keenan, J., Boling, P., Schwartzberg, J., et al. "A National Survey of the Home Visiting Practice and Attitudes of Family Physicians and Internists." *Arch Intern Med* 1992; 152: 2025–32.

30. Steel, K. "Physician-Directed Long-Term Health Care." *J Amer Geriatr Soc* 1987; 35: 264–268.

31. Rossman, I. "The Geriatrician and the Homebound Patient." *J Amer Geriatr Soc* 1988; 36: 348–354.

32. Harris, M. "The Changing Scene in Community Health Nursing." *Nurs Clin N Amer* 1988; 23: 559–568.

33. American Geriatrics Society Policy Committee. "Home Care and Home Care Reimbursement." *J Amer Geriatr Soc* 1989; 37: 1065–66.

34. Fitzgerald, J., Moore, P., Dittus, R. "The Care of Elderly Patients with Hip Fracture. Changes since Implementation of the Prospective Payment System." *N Engl J Med* 1988; 319: 1392–97.

35. Kemp, B., Brummel-Smith, K., Ramsdell, J. *Geriatric Rehabilitation.* Boston: Little, Brown, 1990.

36. Caplan, A., Callahan, D., Haas, J. Ethical and Policy Issues in Rehabilitation Medicine. *Hastings Center Report* 1987 (Special Supplement): 1–20.

37. Sager, M., Easterling, D., Kindig, D., Anderson, O. "Changes in the Location of Death After Passage of Medicare's Prospective Payment System. *N Engl J Med* 1989; 320: 433–439.

38. Gillick, M., Serrell, N., Gillick, L. "Adverse Consequences of Hospitalization in the Elderly." *Soc Sci Med* 1982; 16: 1033–38.

39. Felsenthal, G., Cohen, B., Hilton, E., Panagos, A., Aiken, B. "The Physiatrist on an Inpatient Rehabilitation Unit." *Arch Phys Med Rehab* 1984; 65: 375–378.

40. Johnston, M., Miller, L. "Cost-Effectiveness of the Medicare Three-Hour Regulation." *Arch Phys Med Rehabil* 1986; 67: 581–584.

41. Callahan, J., Wallack, S. *Reforming the Long-Term Care System.* Lexington, MA: Lexington Books, 1981.

42. Harrington, C., Cassel, C., Estes, C., Woolhandler, S., Himmelstein, D., et al. "A National Long-term Care Program for the United States. A Caring Vision." *JAMA* 1991; 266: 3023–29.

43. Ouslander, J., Osterweil, D., and Morley, J. *Medical Care in the Nursing Home.* New York: McGraw-Hill, 1991.

44. Select Committee on Aging. US House of Representatives. American's Elderly at Risk. Publication # 99–508. Washington, D.C.: US GPO 1985.

45. Himmelstein, D., Woolhandler, S. "Cost Without Benefit. Administrative Waste in American Health Care." *N Engl J Med* 1986; 314: 441–445.

46. Berwick, D. "Continuous Improvement as an Ideal in Health Care." *N Engl J Med* 1989; 320: 52–56.

47. 16th Annual Report of the Massachusetts State Board of Lunacy and Charity. *Boston Medical and Surgical J* 1895: 132: 190.

48. May, M., Kaminskas, E., Kasten, J., with Levine, D. *Managing Institutional Long-Term Care for the Elderly.* Gaithersburg, MD: Aspen Publishers, 1991.

49. Batalden, P., Buchanan, E. "Industrial Models of Quality Improvement." In N. Goldfield and D. Nash, eds. *Providing Quality Care.* Philadelphia, PA: American College of Physicians, 1984, pp. 133–159.

50. Vladeck, B. "Quality Assurance Through External Controls." *Inquiry* 1988; 25: 100–107.

51. Donabedian, A. "The Quality of Care: How Can it be Assessed." *JAMA* 1988; 260: 1743–48.

52. Koren, M. "Home Care—Who Cares?" *N Engl J Med* 1986; 314: 917–920.

53. Gray, C. "Quality Assurance in a Rehabilitation Facility—a Decentralized Approach." *Qual Rev Bull* 1988; 14: 9–14.

CONTRIBUTORS

George J. Agich is Professor of Medical Humanities and Psychiatry and Director of the Medical Ethics Program at Southern Illinois School of Medicine. He is author of *Autonomy and Long-Term Care*, and has written on a variety of topics in medical ethics and philosophy of medicine.

David Barnard is Professor and Chair of the Department of Humanities at The Pennsylvania State University College of Medicine. He is a past President of the Society for Health and Human Values and coeditor of *Nourishing the Humanistic in Medicine: Interactions with the Social Sciences.*

Ronald A. Carson is Harris L. Kempner Professor and Director of the Institute for the Medical Humanities, The University of Texas Medical Branch at Galveston. He is a Hastings Center Fellow and coeditor of *Medical Humanities Review.*

Ruthanne L. Curry is a Family Nurse Practitioner in private practice in Gainesville Florida. As the mother of two children, one of whom has a physical disability, she and her husband, Dr. R. Whit Curry, Jr., continue to advocate for integrating all children with differing abilities into community life.

John W. Douard is Assistant Professor in the Institute for the Medical Humanities and in the Department of Preventive Medicine and Community Health, The University of Texas Medical Branch at Galveston.

Sue E. Estroff is Associate Professor in the Department of Social Medicine, School of Medicine, and holds appointments in the departments of Anthropology and Psychiatry at the University of North Carolina at Chapel Hill. She is the author of *Making It Crazy: An Ethnography of Psychiatric Clients in an American Community,* for which she received the Margaret Mead Award from the American Anthropological Association and the Society of Applied Anthropology, as well as numerous articles and essays on persons with severe, persistent mental illness.

Muriel R. Gillick is a physician specializing in geriatrics. She is Assistant Professor of Medicine and the Associate Director of the Geriatrics Fellowship Program at Harvard Medical School. She is the author of *Choosing Medical Care in Old Age: What Kind, How Much, When to Stop,* and of numerous articles on geriatric ethics and health policy.

Arthur Kleinman is Maude and Lillian Presley Professor of Medical Anthropology and Chair of the Department of Social Medicine at Harvard Medical School. He is also Professor of Anthropology at Harvard University and author of numerous works, including *Patients and Healers in the Context of Culture, Rethinking Psychiatry: From Cultural Category to Personal Experience,* and *The Illness Narratives: Suffering, Healing and the Human Condition.*

Lonnie D. Kliever is Professor and Chair of Religious Studies at Southern Methodist University. He is a philosopher of religion interested in the impact of secularization and modernization on religious belief and practice. He was the humanities advisor for the film "Dax's Case," and editor of the companion volume, *Dax's Case: Essays in Medical Ethics and Human Meaning.*

S. Kay Toombs is Assistant Professor of Philosophy at Baylor University. She is the author of *The Meaning of Illness* and numerous articles on the experience of illness, disability, and the phenomenology of the body.

INDEX